Child Welfare Practice with Immigrant Children and Families

Children in immigrant families represent nearly one-fourth of all children living in the United States. As this population of children has increased, so has their representation among children involved in child welfare and related systems. Once immigrant families come to the attention of these systems, they often have multiple and complex needs that must be addressed to ensure children's safety and well-being.

Culturally competent practice with Latino, Asian, and African immigrants requires that professionals understand the impact of immigration and acculturation on immigrant families to conduct adequate assessments and provide interventions that respond appropriately to their needs. Professionals also need to be familiar with federal and state policies that affect immigrant families and how those policies may affect service delivery. At the system level, child welfare agencies need to educate and train a culturally competent workforce that responds appropriately to children and families from diverse cultures.

This book addresses these critical issues and provides recommendations for the development of culturally competent assessment, intervention, and prevention activities in child welfare agencies. This information can be used as a resource by child welfare administrators, practitioners, and students to improve the child welfare system's response to immigrant children and families and promote culturally competent practice.

Part of this book was previously published as a special issue of the *Journal of Public Child Welfare*.

Alan J. Dettlaff is Assistant Professor in the Jane Addams College of Social Work, University of Illinois at Chicago. Prior to entering academia, Dr. Dettlaff practised for several years in public child welfare as a practitioner and administrator, where he specialized in investigations of child maltreatment. Dr. Dettlaff's research interests focus on improving outcomes for children of colour in the child welfare system through the elimination of racial disparities. Dr. Dettlaff is also Principal Investigator of the Jane Addams Child Welfare Training Project, which provides advanced training and financial assistance to students pursuing careers in child welfare.

Rowena Fong is the Ruby Lee Piester Centennial Professor in Services to Children and Families in the School of Social Work at the University of Texas at Austin. She has worked with immigrants in the communities of Boston, San Francisco, Honolulu, and Austin. Her current research is focused on the needs and services available to international and domestic victims of human trafficking. She has over 100 publications and is the author of six books, of which three are about culturally competent practice.

Child Welfare Practice with Immigrant Children and Families

Edited by
Alan J. Dettlaff and Rowena Fong

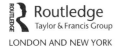

LONDON AND NEW YORK

First published 2012
by Routledge
2 Park Square, Milton Park, Abingdon, Oxfordshire OX14 4RN

Simultaneously published in the USA and Canada
by Routledge
711 Third Avenue, New York, NY 10017

First issued in paperback 2014

Routledge is an imprint of the Taylor and Francis Group, an informa business

British Library Cataloguing in Publication Data
A catalogue record for this book is available from the British Library

ISBN 978-0-415-68469-9 (hbk)
ISBN 978-1-138-79831-1 (pbk)

Typeset in Garamond
by Taylor & Francis Books

Disclaimer
The publisher would like to make readers aware that the chapters in this book are referred to as articles as they had been in the special issue. The publisher accepts responsibility for any inconsistencies that may have arisen in the course of preparing this volume for print.

Contents

Notes on Contributors

Eugene Aisenberg is Associate Professor, University of Washington, School of Social Work, Seattle, WA.

Julie Cooper Altman, Ph.D., is Associate Professor and former Director of the Child Welfare Training Project at the Adelphi University School of Social Work.

Cecilia Ayón is Assistant Professor, Arizona State University, School of Social Work, Phoenix, AZ.

GemJoy Barrett was a Protective Services Specialist at the New York City Administration of Children's Services and a Trainee in the Child Welfare Training Project at the Adelphi University School of Social Work at the time of this study. She is now a writer and small business owner.

Maryellen Bearzi is Administrative Deputy Director, State of New Mexico Children, Youth and Families Department, Santa Fe, NM.

Jenise Brown, M.S.W., was a Protective Services Specialist at the New York City Administration of Children's Services and a Trainee in the Child Welfare Training Project at the Adelphi University School of Social Work at the time of this study. She is now a Supervisor there.

Alma J. Carten is Associate Professor, New York University, Silver School of Social Work, New York, NY.

Luvella Clark-Idusogie, M.S.W., was a Protective Services Specialist at the New York City Administration of Children's Services and a Trainee in the Child Welfare Training Project at the Adelphi University School of Social Work at the time of this study.

Pauline Erera is Associate Professor, University of Washington, School of Social Work, Seattle, WA.

Kya Fawley-King is Postdoctoral Fellow, Child and Adolescent Services Research Center, San Diego, CA.

Jeanne Bertrand Finch is Assistant Dean and Graduate Program Director, Stony Brook University, School of Social Welfare, Stony Brook, NY.

Megan Finno is the former Constituency & Immigration Liaison, State of New Mexico Children, Youth and Families Department, Santa Fe, NM. She is currently a Provost

PhD Fellow in the doctoral program at the University of South California's School of Social Work.

Kathleen Holt is Training and Curriculum Coordinator, University of Kansas, School of Social Welfare, Child Welfare Resource Network, Lawrence, KS.

Robin Leake is Research and Evaluation Manager, Butler Institute for Families, University of Denver, Graduate School of Social Work, Denver, CO.

Yaminah McClendon, M.S.W., was a Protective Services Specialist at the New York City Administration of Children's Services and a Trainee in the Child Welfare Training Project at the Adelphi University School of Social Work at the time of this study. She is currently working as a Child Welfare Social Worker in Great Britain.

Debora M. Ortega is Associate Professor, University of Denver, Graduate School of Social Work, Denver, CO.

Cathryn Potter is Executive Director, Butler Institute for Families, University of Denver, Graduate School of Social Work, Denver, CO.

Sunny Harris Rome is Associate Professor, George Mason University, Department of Social Work, Fairfax, VA.

Tanya Ruiz, M.S.W., was a Protective Services Specialist at the New York City Administration of Children's Services and a Trainee in the Child Welfare Training Project at the Adelphi University School of Social Work at the time of this study.

Chenelle Skepple, M.S.W., was a Protective Services Specialist at the New York City Administration of Children's Services and a Trainee in the Child Welfare Training Project at the Adelphi University School of Social Work at the time of this study.

Latarsha Thomas, M.S.W., was a Protective Services Specialist at the New York City Administration of Children's Services and a Trainee in the Child Welfare Training Project at the Adelphi University School of Social Work at the time of this study. She is now a Supervisor there.

Immigrant Children and Families and Child Welfare

ALAN J. DETTLAFF

This chapter summarizes the literature regarding immigrant children and families in the United States and the challenges they may experience that may make them vulnerable for contact with child welfare systems. The chapter includes a summary of the current state of knowledge regarding immigrant children and families' involvement with child welfare systems and the need for culturally competent child welfare practice with this rapidly increasing population.

Immigrant Children and Families and Child Welfare

Over the past two decades, the demographic profile of the United States has changed considerably as a result of changes in immigration patterns. Not only have the numbers of foreign-born immigrants living in the United States increased, but also a larger proportion of this population consists of children and families. During the 1990s, more than 15 million immigrants entered the United States, an increase of 50% since the 1980s and over 100% since the 1970s (Capps & Fortuny, 2006). As of 2009, 38.5 million of the 307 million residents of the United States were foreign-born immigrants, representing 12.5% of the total U.S. population (Gryn & Larsen, 2010). Along with this growth, the number of children with at least one immigrant parent has more than doubled, from 8 million in 1990 to 16.4 million in 2007 (Fortuny, Capps, Simms, & Chaudry, 2009). Children of immigrants now represent nearly one-fourth (23%) of all children in the United States (Fortuny et al., 2009). More than half (56%) of children of immigrants are of Hispanic origin, while 18% are non-Hispanic white, 18% are non-Hispanic Asian, and 8% are non-Hispanic black (Fortuny & Chaudry, 2009).

Children of immigrants reside primarily in six states that have been traditional destination states for immigrants – California, Texas, New York, Florida, Illinois, and New Jersey. Together, these states account for 67% of all children of immigrants in the United States (Fortuny et al., 2009). However, along with increased immigration flows and changes in immigration patterns, the number of children with immigrant parents has rapidly increased in many western, midwestern, and southeastern states. While the population of children of immigrants grew by 77% in the six destination states from 1990 to 2007, new high-growth states – including North Carolina, Nevada, Georgia, Arkansas, Nebraska, Tennessee, and South Carolina – experienced increases of more than 300% in the population of children of immigrants (Fortuny & Chaudry, 2009).

Although a small number of children of immigrants are foreign-born themselves, most (87%) are U.S. born citizens. However, among children of immigrants, 44% live in families where neither parent is a citizen, and nearly one-third (32%) live in mixed-status families, where the children are citizens, but at least one parent is not (Fortuny & Chaudry, 2009). The share of mixed-status families has increased significantly over the past two decades, increasing from 24% in 1990 to 32% in 2007. Among mixed-status families, significant differences exist by region of origin. In 2007, nearly half (48%) of Mexican children of immigrants lived in mixed-status families, compared to only 14% of European children of immigrants, and 13% of Asian children of immigrants (Fortuny & Chaudry, 2009).

As the population of immigrants has grown, research in child welfare has begun to address issues affecting immigrant children and families. Recent research has documented that children in immigrant families represent approximately 8.6% of all children who come to the attention of child welfare agencies (Dettlaff & Earner, 2010). Although this population is small, immigrant children and families involved in the child welfare system have multiple and complex needs that need to be addressed in order to achieve positive outcomes of safety, permanency, and well-being. Upon migrating to the United States, immigrant families face a multitude of challenges resulting from their experiences with immigration and acculturation. Differences in culture, language, and traditions serve as significant sources of stress for immigrant children and families and create barriers to accessing needed resources. Compounding these stressors are legislative initiatives that restrict immigrant families' access to basic safety net services, affecting even those with legal status. This chapter will review these challenges and their implications for child welfare systems. The chapter will conclude with a review of the current state of knowledge regarding the involvement of immigrant children and families in the child welfare system and introduce the chapters in this text that contribute to our growing understanding of this population.

The Impact of Immigration and Acculturation on Immigrant Children and Families

Children in immigrant families experience unique stresses and pressures that may make them vulnerable to contact with child welfare systems. Literature on families' experiences following immigration cites several sources of risk, including financial challenges, loneliness, isolation, language difficulties, fear, and hopelessness (Earner, 2007; Finno, Vidal de Haymes, & Mindell, 2006; Maiter, Stalker, & Alaggia, 2009). Additional pressures resulting from acculturation can lead to a variety of strains and difficulties on family systems. As a result, child welfare professionals need to understand the impact that immigration and acculturation has on immigrant families in order to provide services that adequately respond to these underlying issues.

The Immigration Experience

While circumstances leading to immigration vary among families, most families choose to migrate because the financial or political situation in their own country has left them with no other options (Segal & Mayadas, 2005). For families living in poverty in their country of origin, the decision to migrate is often based on financial necessity, with families migrating in search of greater wages and increased job opportunities in order to improve the living conditions of the family (Jennissen, 2007). Although reasons for migration vary, the immigration experience represents a major life crisis for most immigrant families that contains both opportunities and risks. Migration may occur in several phases, with family members often migrating in more than one trip until the economic condition in the new country becomes stable enough for all members to join the family (Garcia, 2001). The initial act of entering the country can be very dangerous, with many immigrants experiencing violence, robbery, and sexual assault (Espin, 1987; Solis, 2003). Children are often separated from parents and other siblings for extended periods while placed with family or kin in the country of origin. The stress associated with this initial transition period may result in depression or anxiety, while individuals who experience significant trauma during migration may develop symptoms of post-traumatic stress disorder (Smart & Smart, 1995).

Once in the new country, families continue to experience stress resulting from language barriers, unfamiliar systems, and loss of routine (Hancock, 2005; Solis, 2003). Although many of these challenges are tangible (finding employment, shopping, paying bills, navigating the school and medical systems), each of these challenges can result in significant anxiety and stress. Parents may also struggle to meet the basic needs of their family. Immigrants who are undocumented are likely to experience additional stress, as they live with the ongoing fear of discovery and deportation. As immigration laws become more punitive, these immigrants are at increased risk for discovery and psychological stress. Along with fears of deportation, undocumented parents fear separation from their children, the majority of whom are U.S. citizens (Fortuny et al., 2009). Immigration enforcement activities have increased considerably over the past decade, and have included a number of large, highly publicized worksite raids conducted by Immigration and Customs Enforcement (ICE), the interior enforcement arm of the Department of Homeland Security. In many of these raids, parents were separated from their children for extended periods with no way of contacting them or deported to their country of origin while their children remained in the United States (Capps, Castaneda, Chaudry, & Santos, 2007).

Acculturation and Acculturative Stress

The process of acculturation refers to the internal process of change experienced by all immigrants upon exposure to a new culture (Padilla & Perez, 2003). At the individual level, acculturation involves cultural and psychological changes that occur over a period of time as individuals adapt and respond to a new culture. Acculturative stress is a distinct concept from acculturation, and refers to the stress that directly results from the acculturative process (Berry, Kim, Minde, & Mok, 1987). Upon migration, individuals are faced with a multitude of challenges as they attempt to navigate the new culture. Acculturative stress results when individuals lack the necessary skill or means to interact and be successful in the new environment (Berry et al., 1987). For many immigrants, the acculturative stress experienced following migration is life-long, pervasive, and intense (Smart & Smart, 1995).

Although acculturative stress is supported in the literature among all immigrants, this literature suggests that acculturation is more difficult for those immigrants who are more distinct from the host culture (Leon & Dziegielewski, 1999; Padilla & Perez, 2003). When significant differences exist between the country of origin and the host culture, the process of acculturation becomes more challenging as a result of the cultural negotiation that must occur, as these immigrants must cope with the societal standards and traditions of the new culture, while making decisions about the level to which they will integrate into the host culture. For immigrants of differing religious and cultural backgrounds, this often involves giving up previously valued cultural traditions or feeling pressured to accept certain changes to their traditions.

Thus, immigrants who are more distinct from the host culture in ethnicity, religion, and language are more likely to experience social discrimination and prejudice as a result of the factors that identify them as different from the majority (Padilla & Perez, 2003; Smart & Smart, 1995). Accented speech, unfamiliar customs, and differences in skin color are all factors that identify immigrants as outsiders to those in the new culture. These immigrants may experience additional stress as members of the host culture may question their motives and limit their opportunity for involvement (Padilla & Perez, 2003). When this occurs, some immigrants feel forced to undergo certain changes, rather than choosing the level to which they acculturate, further contributing to stress.

Additionally, the process of moving from an ethnic majority in their country of origin to a minority in the United States can be disorienting for many immigrants from Latin American, Asian, and African countries. While many poor immigrants have experienced discrimination in their country of origin due to their social class, the experience of discrimination for the first time as a result of their ethnicity can add further stress. This transition to minority status combined with the anti-immigrant sentiment that exists in many parts of the United States may result in feelings of stigmatization and isolation for non-white immigrant families. This can lead to feelings of powerlessness and low self-esteem, as immigrants become aware that judgments are made against them based on assumptions of their ethnicity, rather than their actual abilities (Casas, Ponterotto, & Sweeney, 1987).

Risk and Protective Factors in Immigrant Families

In addition to understanding the impact of immigration and acculturation on children and families, child welfare professionals need to understand the resulting challenges and barriers that many immigrant families experience that may make them vulnerable for contact with child welfare systems. In addition to these challenges, federal and state policies intended to limit services or access to resources to only naturalized citizens create further barriers to immigrant children and families' well-being. Yet, despite these challenges, immigrant families possess a number of protective factors that may mitigate against some of this risk. Understanding the risks and protective factors that may be present within immigrant families is necessary to conduct thorough assessments that identify areas of need as well as areas of strength.

Changing Cultural Contexts

Changing cultural contexts can result in multiple sources of family conflict that may increase the risk of maltreatment for children in immigrant families. Following migration, cultural and financial pressures often result in changes to previously established gender roles and expectations (Coltrane, Parke, & Adams, 2004). Financial stressors often necessitate that women enter the workforce, which may require men to accept additional responsibilities for childcare and housework (Coltrane et al., 2004).

Although immigrant women who are employed in the United States generally experience greater autonomy and independence, men may experience the opposite (Pessar, 1999). Research indicates that outside employment of wives and unemployment of men are both significantly associated with domestic violence among immigrant couples (Aldarondo, Kaufman, & Jasinski, 2002; Cunradi, Caetano, & Schafer, 2002). Further, because undocumented immigrants can be deported upon arrest, many cases of domestic violence go unreported as women are afraid of the resulting effects on the family (Aldarondo et al., 2002; Earner, 2010).

Differences in acculturation levels may also produce significant tension between parents who adhere to traditional cultural values and children who adapt more rapidly to the social norms of their new cultural environment (Fontes, 2002; Quinones-Mayo & Dempsey, 2005). Increased parenting stress is common among immigrant parents, who feel they are no longer able to control their children. As parents struggle to maintain discipline, they may become more harsh and rigid in their attempts to regain authority (Bacallao & Smokowski, 2007).

Poverty and Access to Benefits

Immigrant families with children are more likely than U.S. born families to have incomes below the federal poverty level (FPL). In 2008, 21% of immigrant families had incomes below the FPL, compared to 15% of U.S. born families (Chaudry & Fortuny, 2010a). Children of immigrants also were more likely to live in low-income families (defined as family incomes below twice the FPL). Nearly half (49%) of immigrant families were low-income, compared to 35% of U.S. born families (Chaudry & Fortuny, 2010a). Overall, immigrant families are approximately 40% more likely to be poor or low income than U.S. born families. However, significant differences exist among immigrant groups. European, East Asian, and Middle Eastern families have incomes 60% to 80% higher than the mean immigrant family income, while Mexican and Central American families have incomes significantly below the average (Chaudry & Fortuny, 2010a).

Related to the overall lower rates of family income among immigrant families, children in immigrant families are at greater risk than children of U.S. born parents for inadequate nutrition. In 2008, 25% of children of immigrants lived in food-insecure households, compared to 21% of children of U.S. born parents. Children of immigrants are also more likely to live in crowded housing, defined as more than 2 people per bedroom (7% of children of immigrants compared to 2% of children of U.S. born parents) (Chaudry & Fortuny, 2010a). Yet, despite these higher rates of poverty and economic hardship, immigrant families are less likely to receive public benefits (e.g., Temporary Assistance for Needy Families [TANF], Supplemental Nutrition Assistance Progam [SNAP]) (Chaudry & Fortuny, 2010a), and children of immigrants are less likely than children of U.S. born parents to have health insurance (Capps & Fortuny, 2006). These disparities exist largely due to eligibility rules that exclude non-citizen parents, both documented and undocumented, from accessing these benefits even though the majority of children in immigrant families are citizens.

Educational Attainment

Contributing to economic hardship, children in immigrant families are further disadvantaged as a result of parental education. As of 2008, 27% of children of immigrants had parents with less than a high school education, compared to only 7% of children with U.S. born parents (Chaudry & Fortuny, 2010b). Again, significant differences exist according to region of origin, as nearly half (47%) of Mexican children had parents with less than high school educations compared to only 3% to 5% of children of European, East Asian, and Middle Eastern origin (Chaudry & Fortuny, 2010b).

Social Isolation

Migration severs many immigrant families from established support systems in their country of origin and results in the loss of broad networks of extended family (Maiter, Stalker, & Alaggia, 2009). These losses can intensify the stress resulting from acculturation, as families have nobody to turn to in times of need. Anti-immigrant sentiment may increase feelings of isolation and stigmatization. Local community agencies, which could potentially act as extended support systems, may not be accessible to immigrant families due to language barriers or fear of interacting with government or other social service systems. Immigrant parents may also be unfamiliar with how or where to access support from the community.

Parenting Styles and Expectations

Particularly relevant to vulnerability for contact with the child welfare system, differences in parenting styles and expectations may place children in some immigrant families at additional risk. Parenting styles are influenced by a number of factors, including culture, class, education, individual family practices, and personality. For immigrant families, parenting styles are further influenced by their level of acculturation and the unique goals and experiences of each family (Mendez, 2006). Parenting styles are based on cultural practices and attitudes, such as beliefs about the value of punishment and the use of punitive disciplinary strategies to correct behavior. While norms concerning acceptable child rearing and punishment vary by culture, a number of studies have documented the use of authoritarian parenting styles and corporal punishment as a disciplinary strategy prevalent among immigrant parents (Frias-Armenta & McCloskey, 1998; Park, 2001; Tajima & Harachi, 2010). When combined with other stressors such as poverty and acculturative stress, this parenting style may result in harsh physical discipline that can lead to child welfare involvement (Earner, 2007; Rhee, Chang, Weaver, & Wong, 2008).

Differences in parenting expectations may also place immigrant children and families at risk of involvement with child welfare systems. For example, the use of sibling caretaking, in which older children are responsible for the supervision and socialization of younger children, is a common childcare practice in many cultures outside of the United States and among recent immigrants (Hafford, 2010). However, this may be interpreted as neglect or inadequate supervision in the United States depending upon the circumstances and laws of the state (Zielewski, Malm, & Geen, 2006). Similarly, newly arrived immigrant parents who are unfamiliar with U.S. child rearing norms and laws may leave children unattended for short periods, placing them at additional risk for allegations of neglect (Fontes, 2005).

Protective Factors

Despite high levels of economic hardship and other risks, strengths within immigrant family systems as well as their extended networks, may serve as buffers against some of the potential negative consequences resulting from migration. Most important among these may be immigrant families' culture and connections to their countries of origin. Although learning to function in a new culture may serve as a source of stress for many immigrant families, researchers have suggested that adherence to cultural values and beliefs is a significant source of strength that allows individuals to maintain flexibility and cohesion in the face of a changing environment (Falicov, 2005; Hancock, 2005). Additional studies have found that identification with core values and beliefs rooted in their native culture may protect immigrants from experiencing many negative outcomes including substance use and mental health problems (De La Rosa, 2002; Holleran & Waller, 2003).

The presence of two-parent households, a strength of many immigrant families, may provide a family structure that reduces risk for child welfare involvement. In studies examining the incidence of child maltreatment, children living with married biological parents have the lowest overall rates of child abuse and neglect (Sedlak et al., 2010). Children in immigrant families are considerably more likely than children with U.S. born parents to live in two parent households (76% vs. 62%), with children of Middle Eastern and East Asian origin having the highest rates of two-parent families at over 85% (Chaudry & Fortuny, 2010b). Children in immigrant families are also more likely to live in families with three or more adults, including parents and other adult relatives. Extended family members serve as additional sources of support and may provide additional resources for the family system.

Immigrant families' reasons for migration may also serve as a protective factor for their children. Undertaking a long, expensive, and uncertain journey to a foreign country requires determination, strength, and a strong sense of personal and family responsibility. For many immigrant families, the desire for a better life for their children that is often associated with their reasons for migration can be a powerful strength and motivating factor. Additional characteristics often found in immigrant families including strong parental supervision, religious beliefs, and supportive community networks may serve as further protective factors (Dettlaff, Earner, & Phillips, 2009; Harker, 2001).

Immigrant Children and Families Involvement with Child Welfare Systems

As a result of many of the risks associated with immigration and acculturation, children in immigrant families have often been considered at increased risk of maltreatment. Yet, despite this potential vulnerability, very little is known about immigrant families' actual contact and involvement with child welfare systems. This section reviews the current knowledge concerning immigrant families' involvement and experiences with child welfare.

Exact data regarding the number of children in immigrant families who are mal-treated or who come to the attention of child welfare agencies are unknown, as this data is not collected uniformly at the local, state, or national levels. However, recent research has begun to shed some light on this emerging issue. Using data from the National Survey of Child and Adolescent Well-being (NSCAW), a federally-funded and nationally representative survey of children who come to the attention of child welfare agencies, Dettlaff and Earner (2010) found that children living with a foreign-born parent comprise 8.6% of all children who come to the attention of the child welfare system. Among those children, 82.5% are U.S.-born citizens. These data indi-cate that children of immigrants are considerably underrepresented among children who become involved with child welfare agencies, given that children of immigrants represent approximately 23% of the U.S. child population (Fortuny et al., 2009). However, the researchers suggest that it is important to consider reasons that may lead to this underrepresentation. Although this may be an indicator of lower rates of mal-treatment in immigrant families, it is also possible that immigrant families in need of intervention are not coming to the attention of child welfare systems. This could be the result of social isolation, avoidance of social service systems due to concern over immi-gration status, lack of enrollment in school, or lack of access to service providers (Det-tlaff & Earner, 2010).

In addition to identifying the proportion of children in immigrant families among those involved with the child welfare system, this research indicated that certain risk factors associated with maltreatment were significantly more likely to be present in families with U.S. born parents (Dettlaff & Earner, 2010). Specifically, U.S. born par-ents were three times more likely to be actively abusing alcohol or drugs than immi-grant parents and were significantly more likely to have recent histories of arrests. Notably, no significant differences were found in the prevalence of several risk factors often associated with immigrant families, including the use of excessive discipline, active domestic violence, low social support, and difficulty meeting their basic needs (Dettlaff & Earner, 2010). Thus, although immigrant families may face a number of risk factors due to immigration and acculturation, these findings suggest that strengths within immigrant families may serve as buffers against some of these risks.

Concerning the incidence of maltreatment, Dettlaff and Earner (2010) found no significant differences in the overall rates of maltreatment between children in immi-grant families and children in U.S. born families. However, they found that children of immigrants were significantly more likely than children of U.S. born parents to experience emotional abuse. The authors state that interpretation of this finding is difficult as statutory definitions of emotional abuse vary widely across states; however, they suggest that this may be the result of cultural differences in parenting styles or expectations among certain immigrant groups that may be viewed as inappropriate by those unfamiliar with those cultures.

Several additional studies have identified that children in immigrant families may be more vulnerable to certain forms of maltreatment. Among Latino children, several studies have identified higher rates of sexual abuse among children in immigrant families compared to children in U.S. born families. Using data from NSCAW, Dettlaff et al. (2009) found that Latino children of immigrants were more than five times as likely to experience sexual abuse than Latino children of U.S. born parents. Addition-ally, Kuehn, Vericker, and Capps (2007) found that foreign-born Latino children were significantly more likely than U.S. born Latino children to enter foster care because of sexual abuse among children in the Texas child welfare system. Similarly, among undocumented children in the Texas child welfare system, of which 85% are Latino, more than 20% enter foster care due to sexual abuse compared to less than 5% of other children (Center for Public Policy Priorities, 2010). Among children in Asian immigrant families, Chang, Rhee, and Weaver (2006) found that children in immigrant Korean families were more likely to come to the attention of the California child welfare system for physical abuse than children in other ethnic groups, while Rhee et al. (2008) found that children in immigrant Chinese families were more likely to experience physical abuse compared to the general child welfare population. While these studies have begun to shed light on the unique maltreatment patterns and experiences among children in immigrant families, much additional research is needed to fully understand these patterns. This research is necessary in order to develop prevention programs that successfully target immigrant populations.

Advancing Child Welfare Practice with Immigrant Children and Families

Given the complexity of cases involving immigrant children and families, child welfare agencies need to be equipped to effectively respond to their unique needs in order to promote positive outcomes. Culturally competent practice requires that child welfare practitioners understand the impact of migration and acculturation on immigrant families in order to conduct adequate assessments and provide interventions that respond appropriately to their needs. In addition, child welfare practitioners need to be familiar with federal and state policies that affect immigrant children and families and how those policies may affect service delivery. At the system level, child welfare cases involving immigrant families require collaboration between child welfare and human service systems in the U.S. and foreign countries to facilitate positive outcomes. Finally, child welfare systems need to develop mechanisms to recruit and train a bilingual and bicultural workforce that can respond appropriately to children and families from diverse cultures. The chapters in this text address these important considerations and provide recommendations for improving child welfare systems' response to immigrant children and families.

The text begins with a framework for culturally competent child welfare practice by Rowena Fong and Alan J. Dettlaff. Beginning with a review of the literature regarding the challenges immigrant families may face once they become involved with the child welfare system, the chapter then provides a theoretical framework for child welfare practice with immigrant children and families, building on empowerment theory, strengths perspective, the ecological model, and culturally competent practice approaches.

Following this framework is an important chapter by Sunny Harris Rome that addresses the legal barriers faced by non-citizen and unauthorized immigrant families living in the United States and the potentially devastating consequences that deportation poses to mixed status families. The chapter analyzes the Child Citizen Protection Act of 2009, a pending piece of legislation that would allow immigration judges the ability to consider the best interests of citizen children when faced with the potential deportation of a non-citizen parent. The chapter also addresses the role that the public child welfare system plays in ensuring the well-being of children in families that are impacted by immigration enforcement. Understanding the legal issues discussed in this chapter and the fear experienced by many immigrant parents as a result of their immigration status is essential to providing culturally competent services to immigrant families.

Building from this discussion of legal issues, the next two chapters address important practice considerations to facilitate cultural competence when working with immigrant families. In the first, Ayón, Aisenberg, and Erera document the experiences of immigrant Mexican parents involved with the child welfare system. The focus of this chapter is on parents' interactions with their child welfare caseworkers and their experiences in exercising their voice. Based on these experiences, the authors provide timely recommendations for ensuring cultural competence by facilitating parent engagement. Next, Kya Fawley-King addresses the need for culturally competent interventions when working with children in immigrant families in need of mental health services. The chapter reviews the research findings of several evidence-based mental health treatments and assesses their appropriateness for children in immigrant families. The chapter concludes by providing recommendations for ensuring cultural responsiveness when selecting interventions for this population.

The following chapters move to a discussion of child welfare system responses to addressing the needs of immigrant children and families. First, Finno and Bearzi discuss the challenges experienced by immigrant families in the border state of New Mexico and the efforts of this state child welfare system to improve their policies and practices with this population to facilitate positive outcomes. The initiatives described in this chapter can serve as examples of practices for other child welfare systems experiencing changing demographics as a result of a growing immigrant population. Next, Leake, Holt, Potter, and Ortega provide the results of a federally-funded training initiative designed to improve the cultural responsiveness of child welfare staff working with immigrant Latino families in Kansas and Colorado. This unique training model, which incorporates an experiential simulation, provides an example of an innovative strategy to improve the effectiveness of cultural competence training in child welfare agencies.

Finally, the text closes with two chapters that provide examples of innovative educational strategies to prepare the child welfare workforce for practice with immigrant children and families. First, Cooper Altman and colleagues describe a unique MSW training program designed to improve the cultural responsiveness of child welfare practitioners working with immigrant Caribbean families in New York. The program involves an innovative model of knowledge development that is used to inform policy and practice improvements. In the final chapter, Carten and Finch describe an innovative community-based service/educational initiative designed to prepare MSW students for culturally competent preventive practice with immigrant families. Results from the first-year of this initiative are provided along with recommendations for the development of university-agency partnerships.

References

Aldarondo, E., Kaufman, G. K., & Jasinski, J. (2002). A risk marker analysis of wife assault in Latino families. *Violence Against Women, 8,* 429-454.

Bacallao, M. L., & Smokowski, P. R. (2007). The costs of getting ahead: Mexican family system changes after immigration. *Family Relations, 56,* 52-66.

Berry, J. W., Kim, U., Minde, T., & Mok, D. (1987). Comparative studies of acculturative stress. *International Migration Review, 21*, 491-511.

Capps, R., Castaneda, R. M., Chaudry, A., & Santos, R. (2007). *Paying the price: The impact of immigration raids on America's children.* Washington, DC: Urban Institute.

Capps, R., & Fortuny, K. (2006). *Immigration and child and family policy.* Washington, DC: Urban Institute.

Casas, J. M., Ponterotto, J. G., & Sweeney, M. (1987). Stereotyping the stereotyper: A Mexican-American perspective. *Journal of Cross-Cultural Psychology, 18*, 45-57.

Center for Public Policy Priorities. (2010). *Undocumented and abused: A Texas case study of children in the child protective services system.* Austin, TX: Author.

Chang, J., Rhee, S., & Weaver, D. (2006). Characteristics of child abuse in immigrant Korean families and correlates of placement decisions. *Child Abuse & Neglect, 30*, 881-891.

Chaudry, A., & Fortuny, K. (2010a). *Children of immigrants: Economic well-being.* Retrieved from Urban Institute website: http://www.urban.org/publications/412270.html

Chaudry, A., & Fortuny, K. (2010b). *Children of immigrants: Family and parental characteristics.* Retrieved from Urban Institute website: http://www.urban.org/publications/412132.html

Coltrane, S., Parke, R. D., & Adams, M. (2004). Complexity of father involvement in low-income Mexican American families. *Family Relations, 53*, 179-189.

Cunradi, C. B., Caetano, R., & Schafer, J. (2002). Socioeconomic predictors of intimate partner violence among white, black, and Hispanic couples in the United States. *Journal of Family Violence, 17*, 377-389.

De La Rosa, M. (2002). Acculturation and Latino adolescents' substance use: A research agenda for the future. *Substance Use & Misuse, 37*, 429-456.

Dettlaff, A. J., & Earner, I. (2010). *Children of immigrants in the child welfare system: Findings from the National Survey of Child and Adolescent Well-being.* Retrieved from American Humane Association website: http://www.americanhumane.org/protecting-children/programs/child-welfare-migration/

Dettlaff, A. J., Earner, I., & Phillips, S. D. (2009). Latino children of immigrants in the child welfare system: Prevalence, characteristics, and risk. *Children and Youth Services Review, 31*, 775-783.

Earner, I. (2007). Immigrant families and public child welfare: Barriers to services and approaches to change. *Child Welfare, 86*(4), 63-91.

Earner, I. (2010). Double risk: Immigrant mothers, domestic violence and public child welfare services in New York City. *Evaluation and Program Planning, 33*, 288-293.

Espin, O. M. (1987). Psychological impact of migration on Latinas. *Psychology of Women Quarterly, 11*, 489-503.

Falicov, C. J. (2005). Mexican families. In M. McGoldrick, J. Giordano, & N. Garcia-Preto (Eds.), *Ethnicity and family therapy* (3rd ed., pp. 229-241). New York: Guilford Press.

Finno, M., Vidal de Haymes, M., & Mindell, R. (2006). Risk of affective disorders in the migration and acculturation experience of Mexican Americans. *Protecting Children, 21*(2), 22-35.

Fontes, L. A. (2002). Child discipline and physical abuse in immigrant Latino families: Reducing violence and misunderstanding. *Journal of Counseling and Development, 80*, 31-40.

Fontes, L. A. (2005). *Child abuse and culture: Working with diverse families.* New York: Guilford Press.

Fortuny, K., Capps, R., Simms, M., & Chaudry, A. (2009). *Children of immigrants: National and state characteristics.* Retrieved from Urban Institute website: http://www.urban.org/publications/411939.html

Fortuny, K., & Chaudry, A. (2009). *Children of immigrants: Immigration trends.* Retrieved from Urban Institute website: http://www.urban.org/publications/901292.html

Frias-Armenta, M., & McCloskey, L. A. (1998). Determinants of harsh parenting in Mexico. *Journal of Abnormal Child Psychology, 26*, 129-139.

Garcia, E. C. (2001). Parenting in Mexican American families. In N. Boyd Webb (Ed.), *Culturally diverse parent-child and family relationships: A guide for social workers and other practitioners* (pp. 157-180). New York: Columbia University Press.

Gryn, T. A., & Larsen, L. J. (2010). *Nativity status and citizenship in the United States: 2009. American Community Survey Briefs.* Washington, DC: United States Census Bureau.

Hafford, C. (2010). Sibling caretaking in immigrant families: Understanding cultural practices to inform child welfare practice and evaluation. *Evaluation and Program Planning, 33,* 294-302.

Hancock, T. U. (2005). Cultural competence in the assessment of poor Mexican families in the rural southeastern United States. *Child Welfare, 84,* 689-711.

Harker, K. (2001). Immigrant generation, assimilation, and adolescent psychological well-being. *Social Forces, 79,* 969-1004.

Holleran, L. K., & Waller, M. A. (2003). Sources of resilience among Chicano/a youth: Forging identities in the borderlands. *Child and Adolescent Social Work, 20,* 335-350.

Jennissen, R. (2007). Causality chains in the international migration systems approach. *Population Research and Policy Review, 26,* 411-436.

Kuehn, D., Vericker, T., & Capps, R. (2007). *Child sexual abuse: Removals by child generation and ethnicity.* Retrieved from Urban Institute website: http://www.urban.org/publications /311460.html

Leon, A. M., & Dziegielewski, S. F. (1999). The psychological impact of migration: Practice considerations in working with Hispanic women. *Journal of Social Work Practice, 13*(1), 69-82.

Maiter, S., Stalker, C. A., & Alaggia, R. (2009). The experiences of minority immigrant families receiving child welfare services: Seeking to understand how to reduce risk and increase protective factors. *Families in Society, 90,* 28-36.

Mendez, J. A. O. (2006). Latino parenting expectations and styles: A literature review. *Protecting Children, 21*(2), 53-61.

Padilla, A. M., & Perez, W. (2003). Acculturation, social identity, and social cognition: A new perspective. *Hispanic Journal of Behavioral Sciences, 25,* 35-55.

Park, M. S. (2001). The factors of child physical abuse in Korean immigrant families. *Child Abuse & Neglect, 25,* 945-958.

Pessar, P. R. (1999). Engendering migration studies: The case of new immigrants in the United States. *American Behavioral Scientist, 42,* 577-600.

Quinones-Mayo, Y., & Dempsey, P. (2005). Finding the bicultural balance: Immigrant Latino mothers raising "American" adolescents. *Child Welfare, 84*(5), 649-667.

Rhee, S., Chang, J., Weaver, D., & Wong, D. (2008). Child maltreatment among immigrant Chinese families: Characteristics and patterns of placement. *Child Maltreatment, 13,* 269-279.

Sedlak, A. J., Mettenburg, J., Basena, M., Petta, I., McPherson, K., Greene, A., & Li, S. (2010). *Fourth National Incidence Study of Child Abuse and Neglect (NIS–4): Report to Congress.* Washington, DC: U.S. Department of Health and Human Services, Administration for Children and Families.

Segal, U., & Mayadas, N. (2005). Assessment of issues facing immigrant and refugee families. *Child Welfare, 84,* 563-583.

Smart, J. F., & Smart, D. W. (1995). Acculturative stress of Hispanics: Loss and challenge. *Journal of Counseling and Development, 73,* 390-396.

Solis, J. (2003). Re-thinking illegality as a violence against, not by Mexican immigrants, children, and youth. *Journal of Social Issues, 59,* 15-31.

Tajima, E. A., & Harachi, T. W. (2010). Parenting beliefs and physical discipline practices among southeast Asian immigrants: Parenting in the context of cultural adaptation to the United States. *Journal of Cross-Cultural Psychology, 41,* 212-235.

Zielewski, E. R., Malm, K., & Geen, R. (2006). Children caring for themselves and child neglect: When do they overlap? Washington, DC: Urban Institute.

Culturally Competent Practice with Immigrant Children and Families in Child Welfare

ROWENA FONG and ALAN J. DETTLAFF

This chapter provides an overview of the challenges immigrant children and families may face once they become involved with the child welfare system. The chapter then provides a theoretical framework for child welfare practice with immigrant children and families, building on concepts from empowerment theory, the strengths perspective, the ecological model, and culturally competent practice approaches.

Culturally Competent Practice with Immigrant Children and Families in Child Welfare

One out of ten persons in the United States is foreign born (Gryn & Larsen, 2010) and nearly one out of four children (23%) in the United States has at least one immigrant parent (Fortuny, Capps, Simms, & Chaudry, 2009). The demographics in the United States are changing rapidly but the services for immigrant and ethnic minority children and families in social service systems, such as the public child welfare system, are not.

The stressors for immigrant children and families are similar to those for clients who are American-born; however, as stated in Chapter One, immigrant children and families experience additional pressures. As the first chapter notes, foreign-born Latino children were more likely than U.S.-born Latino children to suffer sexual abuse in the public child welfare system, specifically in Texas (Kuehn, Vericker, & Capps 2007). How does a public child welfare worker discern whether the stressors for a foreign-born Latino child are different from those experienced by a U.S. born Latino child?

This question indicates that, in addition to the individual histories of their migration journeys and perhaps trauma experiences of their foreign-born clients, child welfare case workers need to know about the cultural differences between their foreign- and American-born clients in terms of values, norms and stressors. Very few studies have examined what happens to these immigrant children and families in child welfare systems. These studies indicate that the likelihood of positive outcomes is diminished by poverty, limited access to benefits, fewer sources of social support, differing language and cultural norms, distrust of government, and fear of deportation (Earner, 2007; 2010). Immigrant families may also experience different service paths depending on their documentation status and language abilities (Ayón, 2009), their child's generation in the United States (Vericker, Kuehn, & Capps, 2007), and their race/ethnicity (Rajendran & Chemtob, 2010).

Challenges and Outcomes of Children in Immigrant Families in Child Welfare

The goal of the child welfare system is to ensure the safety, permanency, and well-being of children who come to the attention of this system. Despite the lack of empirical evidence examining outcomes for immigrant children and families, it is clear that immigrant families face a number of challenges that may impede service delivery and positive outcomes, particularly when it is necessary for children to enter substitute care. When children are maltreated in their homes, it is sometimes necessary for their safety and well-being to remove and place them in substitute care. In these instances, substitute care is always a temporary solution, and the goal is to facilitate permanency for the children while ensuring their ongoing safety and well-being. Permanency is best achieved when children are reunited with their parents following services that reduce the risk of maltreatment or otherwise resolve the conditions that warranted removal. Yet, when these children enter substitute care, they may face challenges that threaten the system's ability to facilitate reunification, as well as positive outcomes related to their health and well-being.

Achieving reunification largely depends on the child welfare system's ability to provide family services that reduce the risk factors associated with maltreatment in the home, as well as the parents' meaningful participation and engagement in these services. Yet, if caseworkers fail to discern and address cultural factors in their assessment of families' service needs, their cultural biases or misunderstandings can affect service delivery (Earner, 2007). Cultural values shape the ways in which families view their problems, accept responsibility, and respond to interventions. Failing to understand these elements has, in fact, been cited as the primary barrier to adequate assessment and effective intervention in cases of child maltreatment among immigrant families (Shor, 1999). Thus, the accuracy of assessments and the effectiveness of intervention recommendations for immigrant families both depend on the accuracy of the caseworker's insights into the families' cultural backgrounds and how culture and child-rearing traditions influence their thoughts and actions.

Of additional concern for immigrant children and families is access to services in their preferred language, which is a challenge for many child welfare systems (Ayón, 2009; Barrios, Suleiman, & Vidal de Haymes, 2004). Language barriers can cause miscommunication and misunderstandings that, in turn, can diminish families' ability and motivation to respond positively to interventions. Language barriers create delays in service delivery and impede parents' abilities to complete required services. Such delays may place them at risk for termination of parental rights due to the timeframes mandated by the Adoption and Safe Families Act (ASFA) of 1997 (Ayón, 2009; Committee for Hispanic Children and Families, 2003). ASFA calls for permanency decisions to be made in 12 months, and requires that petitions for termination of parental rights be filed for children who have been in substitute care for 15 of the last 22 months. This has accelerated child welfare case proceedings and instigated more terminations of parental rights and adoptions. Without accessible services in their native languages, the expedited process may pose a considerable threat to meeting case requirements, placing the parents at greater risk of having their parental rights terminated.

For immigrant children in substitute care, the lack of culturally or linguistically appropriate services can also limit their ability to receive services needed to address both the physical and mental health issues resulting from maltreatment (Dettlaff & Cardoso, 2010). Further, funding for immigrant children's services may be limited due to restrictions within Title IV-E of the Social Security Act, which serves as the primary source of federal child welfare funding to states. This funding source allows states to receive federal matching funds for the care of children in state custody. However, the receipt of Title IV-E funds is restricted to children who meet eligibility requirements, including immigration status. Since undocumented immigrant children do not meet the eligibility requirement, the states must bear the total burden of the cost of their substitute care. In times of shrinking resources for public child welfare systems, this may limit states' abilities to adequately care for these children.

In cases where reunification is not possible, adoption or placement with relatives are permanency options. Most importantly, when reunification is not possible, undocumented immigrant children may be eligible for Special Immigrant Juvenile Status (SIJS), which makes them immediately eligible to apply for legal permanent residency in the United States. This status is available for undocumented children under the jurisdiction of a court due to dependency or delinquency. With this status, immigrant children become Title IV-E eligible, and receive the other benefits of legal permanent residency, including the ability to live and work permanently in the United States. However, as SIJS is only available to children for whom reunification with their parents is not an option, the pursuit of SIJS must be done only after determining that reunification or placement with relatives in their country of origin is not in their best interest (Lincroft & Cervantes, 2010).

Finally, lack of collaboration between the U.S. and foreign countries may further restrict families' access to timely and necessary services. Many child welfare cases involving immigrant families have transnational dimensions that require collaboration between child welfare and human service systems in both the sending and receiving countries (e.g., obtaining birth certificates from the country of origin, obtaining home studies by local child welfare authorities for transnational family placements, and obtaining documentation needed to complete applications for immigration relief). However, such collaboration and coordination between most states and foreign countries is rare.

Need for Culturally Competent Practices in Child Welfare

Although child abuse and neglect, domestic violence, substance abuse, and runaway youth may be common in child welfare caseloads, the child welfare caseworker's approach to handling the problems with immigrant children and families is enhanced through culturally competent practice. Delgado, Jones, and Rohani (2005) assert that in working with immigrant newcomer youth who may be "at risk" for failure in this society, "cultural competence serves to ensure that the backgrounds of the youth are not lost in the process of assessing their assets, needs, goals, and it serves as a basis from which to implement youth development guided interventions" (p. 149). Culturally competent practice is also advantageous when child welfare workers arrange for transnational family placements or substitute care that supports the cultural values and traditions in which immigrant children were raised, or using language-appropriate interpreters in family group conferencing with non-English speaking families.

In working with children and youth, Brissett-Chapman (2000) reiterates the benefits for culturally competent practices in placing children in out-of-home care in child welfare. She asks, "How do I help children maintain cultural identity when they are placed in out-of-home care?" and responds by saying, culturally competent organizations are most effective in supporting out-of-home placement due to their recognition of the need to recognize the cultural and ethnic diversity of the client population the agency serves.

Indeed, the organization's policymakers or governing boards ensure a process for developing and updating a mission that reflects a commitment to the population served, recruiting diverse staff, and evaluating policy and program directions with input from individuals from the different cultures or ethnic groups.

The importance of cultural identity for all clients is valued. Children who are placed in out-of-home care require a program that engages its staff and non-relative caregivers in training regarding cross cultural communication, culturally diverse family customs, and conflict resolution (p. 426).

Obtaining training and receiving additional knowledge about culturally diverse family customs, values, and beliefs are key to cultural competence with immigrant children and families. Culturally competent child welfare workers possess cross-cultural knowledge, understand ethnic cultural values, and use culturally appropriate skills in making assessments and recommending services for immigrant children and families in the child welfare system.

Culturally Competent Practices in Working with Immigrant Children and Families

Cultural competence has been a concept familiar to the human service fields for thirty years (Delgado, Jones, & Rahani, 2005). Cultural competence is grounded on the concept of culture, which according to Locke (1992), "is the body of learned beliefs, traditions, principles, and guides for behavior that are commonly shared among members of a particular group. Culture serves as a road map for both perceiving and interacting with the world" (p.10).

Cultural competency encompasses four areas: 1) cultural awareness, 2) knowledge acquisition, 3) skill development, and 4) inductive learning (Lum, 2011). As this list implies, competence extends beyond understanding the immigrant clients' cultural values and using them in making assessments. Cultural competence in social work also entails familiarity with indigenous treatments and using them in intervention planning and implementation, and using cultural values as strengths in both assessments and interventions (Fong & Furuto, 2001; Fong, 2011).

While the need for culturally competent practice when working with immigrant children and families may be widely acknowledged, it remains underutilized or is not fully developed in child welfare worker training programs. Leake, Holt, Potter & Ortega (2010) state that "most cultural responsive trainings available to child welfare professionals focus on acquiring knowledge about a particular cultural group. This, coupled with the desire of workers to have a 'recipe card' approach to understanding complex features can foster false assumptions or stereotypes related to language, religious affiliation, immigration status, and citizenship" (p.327). False assumptions, racial biases, and discriminatory practices are neither what vulnerable clients in the child welfare system need nor deserve to experience. The National Association of Social Work (2001) adopted Cultural Competence Standards in Social Work Practice that emphasize the important of providing culturally competent practice and provide guidance to social workers practicing with diverse clients. According to Standard Three–Cross Cultural Knowledge, "Social Workers shall have and continue to develop specialized knowledge and understanding about the history, traditions, values, family systems, and artistic expressions of major client groups they serve" (p. 4). Standard Four – Cross Cultural Skills stipulates that, "Social workers shall use appropriate methodological approaches, skills, and techniques that reflect the workers' understanding of the role of culture in the helping process" (p. 4).

Recognizing the need for improvements in child welfare agencies' responses to immigrant families, Dettlaff (2008) developed a framework for conducting culturally competent assessments of Latino immigrant children and families involved in the child welfare system. The framework was designed to provide social workers with the information necessary to understand the impact of migration and acculturation immigrant families and the extent to which issues of child maltreatment are related to acculturative stress, cultural conflict, and lack of environmental resources and supports. The framework also provides the opportunity to gather information concerning family strengths, which are often embedded in families' cultural values and traditions.

Theoretical Frameworks to Guide Culturally Competent Practices

The theoretical frameworks in which to use cultural knowledge and skills with immigrant parents and children are essential supports to good practice. Theoretical frameworks not only guide helping professionals in approaching and understanding clients, but help them make decisions about the problem situations which require treatment. Operating within their clients' theoretical frameworks allows professionals to engage clients directly in a working relationship. In working with immigrant children and families, three theoretical frameworks have been especially helpful: strengths perspective, ecological model, and empowerment theory.

Strengths Perspective

The strengths perspective (Saleeby, 2008) is a theory that assumes that everyone has positive characteristics and skills that enhance his or her well-being and functioning. These strengths can be individual characteristics such as intelligence, articulateness, or reliability. Skill areas such as having the ability to facilitate meetings, building houses, or negotiating contracts are other indicators of personal strengths. These strengths are also evident at several levels: the micro level of the individual, the mezzo level of the family, and the macro level of a society.

Strengths from family systems and within family members are included in the positive resources to child welfare clients. Yet another form of strengths that are available to immigrant families is cultural values and norms. Cultural values and norms are beliefs that guide expectations in the attitudes and behaviors of persons who belong to that cultural or racial group. These cultural values are protective factors in most case but can also be risk factors in other cases. For Latino immigrant children and families, it is known that the cultural value of family (*familismo*) is very important. So in working with this population, including family members should be a normal practice of the child welfare caseworker. Furman and Negi (2010) write in their book on *Social Work Practice with Latinos* that the use of family conferencing in child welfare is a culturally responsive intervention.

Often in working with clients in public child welfare the strengths of the parent or family are ignored or forgotten because attention is fixed on the maltreatment problem. A neglectful parent is often perceived as being totally irresponsible for not providing adequate food or supervision for the child, but that neglectful parent's strength in providing for the child emotionally or in other ways may not be acknowledged. Undocumented immigrant parents tend to be viewed negatively because of their immigration status and not because of their parenting ability.

Ayon, Aisenberg, and Erera (2010) warn, "By labeling parents as unfit, the child welfare system challenges the core values of Mexican families and their parenting. This factor alone may impact how parents interact with their worker" (p. 268). Misunderstandings can be avoided if a child welfare worker adopts a strengths perspective toward the family and understands more about their backgrounds and migration journeys.

Ecological Model

The ecological model is a means to understanding people in their social environments and is based on the premise that when people change social environments they also change the ways they behave. The theory advocates taking multiple perspectives of an individual (or group) and not a single view that may be biased or poorly informed. Browne and Mills (2001) assert that the ecological perspective is not a model or theory but a paradigm shift in how one looks at and approaches practice. Person-in-environment, based on the science of human ecology, is a perspective often associated with the ecological model (Germain & Gitterman, 1995). Child welfare workers guided by these approaches need to ask what the client immigrant family was like in their country of origin environment before coming to the United States, or what the physical or social or political environment was like when the immigrant traveled from their country of origin to the United States.

An easily over-looked aspect of the social environment is the migration journey children and families have experienced, and anyone working with immigrants should be alert to the significance of the event. The journey may have involved stressful environments or traumatic events that continue to color their perspectives and responses for months and years after. For example, Ayon, Aisenberg and Erera (2010) write about the experiences of new immigrant Mexican families, who are likely to be fearful of their interactions with public systems, such as the child welfare system, since such contacts could lead to deportation.

Fully understanding the social environment is also a step toward making accurate and culturally competent assessments that allow for clients to get appropriate help, realize their potential, and empower themselves. This last is the focus of empowerment theory.

Empowerment Theory

Empowering people is part of the core mission of the social work profession and empowerment theory operates on the premise that people, when offered the needed assistance, can realize their potential. Empowerment can occur with individuals, communities, and societies. Browne and Mills (2001) refer to Browne's (1995) analysis of empowerment as an intervention, a process, and a skill. Gutierrez (1990) wrote about the empowerment of women of color and Browne and Mills (2001) restate Gutierrez's work, "Women [of color] who were assisted in helping others developed enhanced capabilities" (p. 23).

The empowerment approach offsets the powerlessness felt and or experienced by some oppressed groups of people. One of the principles of the empowerment approach states, "Powerless individuals, groups, and communities, are sometimes stigmatized. Usually consumers are powerless based on their ethnicity, gender, religion, affiliation, sexual orientation, and/or physical and mental status" (Furuto, 2004, p. 29).

Immigrant women, children, and families are likely to experience different forms of powerlessness during their transition and acculturation to the United States. Empowerment would be a very important goal for child welfare workers to identify in their short-term or long-term case plans for immigrant families. Having culturally competent assessments and treatments by using a strengths perspective, person-in-environment, and empowerment approach would facilitate the process of reaching this goal.

References

Ayón, C. (2009). Shorter time-lines, yet higher hurdles: Mexican families' access to child welfare mandated services. *Children and Youth Services Review, 31,* 609-616.

Ayon, C., Aisenberg, E. & Erera, P. (2010). Learning how to dance with the public child welfare system: Mexican parents' efforts to exercise their voice. *Journal of Public Child Welfare,* Vol. 4, No. 3, 263-286.

Barrios, L., Suleiman, L., & Vidal de Haymes, M. (2004). Latino population trends and child welfare services: Reflections on policy, practice, and research from the Latino Consortium roundtable discussions. *Illinois Child Welfare, 1,* 106-114.

Brissett-Chapman, S. (2000) How do I help children adjust to out-of-home care. In H. Dubowitz & D. DePanfilis. (Eds). *Handbook for child protection practice.* pp. 425-430. Thousand Oaks, CA: Sage Publisher.

Browne, C. (1995). Empowerment in social work practice with older women. *Social Work,* 40, 358-364.

Browne, C. & Mills, C. (2001). Theoretical frameworks: Ecological model, strengths perspective and empowerment theory. In R. Fong & S. Furuto (Ed.). *Culturally competent practice: Skills, interventions, and evaluations.* pp. 10-32. Bosotn, MA: Allyn and Bacon.

Committee for Hispanic Children and Families. (2003). *Creating a Latino child welfare agenda: A strategic framework for change.* New York, NY: Author.

Delgado, M., Jones, K., & Rohani, M. (2005). *Social work practice with refugee and immigrant youth.* Boston, MA: Allyn and Bacon.

Dettlaff, A. J. (2008). Immigrant Latino children and families in child welfare: A framework for conducting a cultural assessment. *Journal of Public Child Welfare, 2,* 451-470.

Dettlaff, A. J., & Cardoso, J. B. (2010). Mental health need and service use among Latino children of immigrants in the child welfare system. *Children and Youth Services Review, 32,* 1373-1379.

Earner, I. (2007). Immigrant families and public child welfare: Barriers to services and approaches to change. *Child Welfare,* 86(4), 63-91.

Earner, I. (2010). Double risk: Immigrant mothers, domestic violence and public child welfare services in New York City. *Evaluation and Program Planning, 33,* 288-293.

Fong, R. & Furuto, S. (Eds.). (2001). *Culturally competent practice: Skills, interventions, and evaluations.* Boston, MA: Allyn and Bacon.

Fong, R. (2011). Cultural competence with Asian Americans. In D. Lum (Ed.). *Culturally competent practice: A framework for understanding diverse groups and justice issues.* pp. 333-357. Belmont, CA: Brooks/Cole.

Fortuny, K., Capps, R., Simms, M., & Chaudry, A. (2009). *Children of immigrants: National and state characteristics.* Retrieved from Urban Institute website: http://www.urban.org/publications/411939.html

Furman, R. & Negi, Nalini. (2010). *Social work practice with Latinos.* New York: Lyceum Books.

Furuto, S. (2004). Theoretical perspectives for culturally competent practice with immigrant children and families. In R. Fong (Ed.). *Culturally competent practice with immigrant and refugee children and families.* pp. 19-38. New York: The Guilford Press.

Germain, C. & Gitterman, A. (1995). Ecological perspective. In National Association of Social Workers. (Ed.). *19th encyclopedia of social work.* Vol. 1. Washington, D.C.: NASW Press.

Gryn, T. A., & Larsen, L. J. (2010). *Nativity status and citizenship in the United States: 2009. American Community Survey Briefs.* Washington, DC: United States Census Bureau.

Gutierrez, L. (1990). Working with women of color. *Social Work, 35,* 149-154.

Kuehn, D., Vericker, T., & Capps, R. (2007). *Child sexual abuse: Removals by child generation and ethnicity.* Retrieved from Urban Institute website: http://www.urban.org/publications/311460.html

Leake, R., Holt, K., Potter, C., & Ortega, D. (2010). Using simulation training to improve culturally responsive social work practice. *Journal of Public Child Welfare.* Vol. 4, No. 2, 325-346.

Lincroft, Y., & Cervantes, W. (2010). *Language, culture, and immigration relief options.* Washington, DC: First Focus.

Locke, D. (1992). *Increasing multicultural understanding: A comprehensive model.* Newbury Park, CA: Sage.

Lum, D. (Ed.) (2011).*Culturally competent practice: A framework for understanding* diverse groups and justice issues. Belmont, CA: Brooks/Cole.

National Association of Social Work (2001). *NASW Standards for Cultural Competence in Social Work Practice.* Washington DC: NASW Press.

Rajendran, K., & Chemtob, C. M. (2010). Factors associated with service use among immigrants in the child welfare system. *Evaluation and Program Planning, 33,* 317-323.

Saleeby, D. (2008). *The strengths perspective in social work practice.* 5th ed. Boston, MA: Allyn and Bacon.

Shor, R. (1999). Inappropriate child rearing practices as perceived by Jewish immigrant parents from the former Soviet Union. *Child Abuse & Neglect, 23,* 487-499.

Vericker, T., Kuehn, D. and Capps, R. (2007). Latino children of immigrants in the Texas child welfare system. *Protecting Children, 22(2),* 20-40.

Promoting Family Integrity:
The Child Citizen Protection Act and its
Implications for Public Child Welfare

SUNNY HARRIS ROME

Family integrity, although central to child welfare, is undermined by immigration laws that fail to consider the best interests of the child. This article discusses the threat that deportation poses to family integrity and analyzes the Child Citizen Protection Act of 2009, a potential remedy pending before the United States Congress. It also addresses the roles that public child welfare agencies can play to ensure the well-being of children in mixed-status immigrant families.

Family unification has long been a goal of both American immigration law and child welfare policy. In child welfare, the priority is on keeping families safely together whenever possible. The Adoption Assistance and Child Welfare Act of 1980 (P.L. 96-272) promotes family unification and reunification by requiring states to make "reasonable efforts" to prevent the removal of children from home and, if removed, to return children home as quickly as possible. The Family Preservation and Support Services Program Act of 1993 (P.L. 103-66) provides financial incentives for states to provide intensive family preservation and family support services, both designed to avoid unnecessary removal of children from home. While the Adoption and Safe Families Act of 1997 (P.L. 105-89) focuses on the primacy of child safety and shortens the allowable time for making permanent placements, the Fostering Connections to Success and Increasing Adoptions Act of 2008 (P.L. 110-351) gives states additional tools to link children with relative caregivers.

Since 1965, American immigration law has also prioritized family unification. The Immigration and Nationality Act of 1965 (P.L. 89-236) initiated a system, still in force today, that gives preference to relatives of immigrants already in the United States. Under current law, immediate relatives (spouses, minor children, and parents of adult American citizens) are entitled to apply for legal status without a waiting period, while other eligible relatives receive a priority date based on their preference category and their country of origin. Family-sponsored immigration is the largest source of legal immigration to the United States, accounting for approximately 65% of new legal permanent residents (Monger & Rytina, 2009). Family unification is relied on especially heavily by applicants from the Dominican Republic, Mexico, Jamaica, Columbia, and the Philippines, where it is the basis for more than 75% of each country's total immigration to the United States (McKay, 2003).

The principle of keeping families together is also central to international agreements on human rights, including the Universal Declaration of Human Rights and the International Covenant on Civil and Political Rights (Human Rights Watch, 2007). Unfortunately, despite the fact that American child welfare and immigration policy both purport to value family unity, other aspects of American law subvert family integrity and undermine the best interests of the child when it comes to noncitizen families. Under the Personal Responsibility and Work Opportunity Reconciliation Act of 1996 (P.L. 104-193), for example, undocumented immigrants are ineligible for most federal benefit programs including food stamps, Supplemental Security Income (SSI), Temporary Assistance for Needy Families (TANF), non-emergency Medicaid, and State Children's Health Insurance Program (SCHIP), whereas most legal permanent residents ("green card" holders) are subject to a 5-year waiting period. These benefit restrictions create a hardship for children in immigrant families, who are disproportionately poor and more likely than children in native families to lack health insurance, live in overcrowded housing, and experience food insecurity (Capps, 2008). Additional risk stems from immigrant parents' lower levels of educational achievement, higher unemployment rates, limited English proficiency, and linguistic isolation (Passel & Cohn, 2009). Compounded by lack of access to federal financial assistance, these vulnerabilities may impede the ability of parents to provide a safe and stable environment for their children, increasing the likelihood of separation and reducing the likelihood of reunification (Borelli, Earner, & Lincroft, 2007; Rome, 2008).

Work site raids and other enforcement actions comprise another threat to family integrity. In keeping with its unabashedly aggressive strategy, Immigration and Customs Enforcement (ICE) conducted a record number of raids during the Bush administration; they skyrocketed from approximately 500 in 2005 to more than 1,000 in 2006 (Dettlaff & Phillips, 2007). In 2007, these raids resulted in approximately 5,000 arrests, most for non-criminal conduct (United States Immigration and Customs Enforcement, 2007). The effects of these raids on young children have been well documented. Some were stranded at school or in day care, and others left unsupervised, bewildered, and frightened while their parents were processed and detained (Capps, Castaneda, Chaudry, & Santos, 2007). Beyond the immediate trauma, there is evidence of long-term detrimental consequences:

> Psychologists, teachers, and family members have reported significant increases in instances of anxiety, depression, feelings of abandonment, eating and sleeping disorders, post-traumatic stress disorder, and behavioral changes among children who have experienced the loss of a loved one or who witnessed ICE in action. (Kremer, Moccio, & Hammell, 2009)

Of course, the ultimate threat to family integrity is *deportation*, now termed *removal*. As noted by Thronson (2006), "Although the role of family is critical in shaping who qualifies to immigrate to the United States, when a person faces removal from the United States, it is as an individual, not as a family unit" (p. 1188). For mixed-status families, estimated to include approximately 4 million United States-born children with at least one noncitizen parent, the prospect of deportation is devastating. In these families, where the children remain legally entitled to citizenship in the United States, a parent's deportation poses a Catch-22: either the children exercise their rights, remain in the country, and suffer the tragedy of separation from their parents—or they relinquish their legal rights, their home, and often the only life they know to face potentially hazardous conditions in an unfamiliar country. This article discusses the threat that deportation poses to family integrity and analyzes the Child Citizen Protection Act of 2009, a potential remedy pending in the United States Congress. It also addresses the roles that public child welfare can and should play in ensuring the well-being of children in immigrant families.

Throughout this article, the terms *unauthorized immigrant* and *undocumented immigrant* are used interchangeably. Both terms refer to noncitizens lacking legal permanent residency status, most of whom either entered the country without authorization or overstayed legal visas. Similarly, the terms deportation and removal are used interchangeably to refer to residents compelled by immigration authorities to leave the country; the former term was replaced by the latter in the mid-1990s.

DEPORTATION UNDER CURRENT LAW

Two laws enacted in 1996, the Illegal Immigration Reform and Immigrant Responsibility Act (IIRIRA) and the Antiterrorism and Effective Death Penalty Act (AEDPA), had the effect of drastically altering American deportation policy. Together, they significantly increased the likelihood of family separation by expanding the circumstances under which noncitizens can be removed, limiting judicial discretion, and restricting opportunities for relief.

Under current law, those who enter the country without authorization are subject to deportation. Once deported, they are prohibited from returning to the United States for up to 10 years. In addition, so-called "legal" or "documented" immigrants are subject to mandatory deportation if they commit an "aggravated felony." Contrary to what the term *aggravated felony* would suggest, these acts are neither limited to the most egregious crimes nor are they necessarily felonies. Aggravated felonies include drug offenses, traffic offenses, assault, larceny, weapons violations, forgery, invasion of privacy, liquor violations, tax evasion, obstruction of justice, gambling, threats, obscenity, and others, many of which qualify as misdemeanors under state law. Relatively few immigrants are deported for serious, violent crimes, while examples abound of immigrants being removed for comparatively minor, non-violent offenses including shoplifting, forging checks, marijuana possession, disorderly conduct, and unauthorized use of a vehicle. According to Human Rights Watch (2007), 64.6% of deportations in 2005 were for non-violent offenses, while only 20.9% were for violent offenses and 14.7% were for "other crimes." Similarly, between 1997 and 2007, an estimated 72% of deportations were for non-violent offenses while 27.8% were for violent or potentially violent offenses (only 14% of which involved violence against persons). The most common offenses underlying deportation were: entering the United States illegally (24%), driving under the influence (7.2%), assault (5.5%), and falsifying immigration documents (5.5%). By comparison, robbery accounted for 2.2% of removals, aggravated assault for 1%, and homicide for 0.3% (Human Rights Watch, 2009). Once removed, aggravated felons are permanently barred from reentering the United States (Office of Inspector General, 2009). Furthermore, the law can be applied retroactively; that is, even if a legal permanent resident committed an offense before the law was in effect and has lived peacefully and productively in the United States for decades, that resident can nonetheless be apprehended and deported. This broadly expanded definition of the crimes that render an immigrant subject to mandatory deportation belies common sense and runs contrary to the public's understanding. Lives are ruined and families torn apart, in many cases because of offenses committed long ago and considered under state law to be minor. Estimates suggest that the 897,099 deportations on criminal grounds that occurred between 1997 and 2007 left more than 1 million spouses and children (including American citizens and legal permanent residents) separated from their loved ones (Human Rights Watch, 2009).

From the 1950s to the 1990s, the law provided noncitizens with a range of opportunities to defend against deportation. Most have since been eliminated. Up until 1996, legal permanent residents who had lived in the United States for at least 7 years and were facing deportation were entitled to a hearing, during which the judge would balance mitigating factors against those weighing in favor of deportation. Among the positive considerations were:

- family ties in the United States;
- residence in the United States for a long time or having entered the country as a child;
- service in the United States military;
- an employment history;
- property or business ties in the United States;
- making valuable contributions to the community;
- providing evidence of good character or proof of rehabilitation; and
- showing that deportation would cause hardship to oneself or one's family (Immigration and Nationality Act, 1952).

These hearings allowed judges to exercise discretion on a case-by-case basis. Instead, current law mandates deportation using one-size-fits-all criteria that fail to take an immigrant's background, contributions, and family situation into account. This policy is at odds with the European Union, where judges must consider an immigrant's duration of residence, age, connection to the expelling and receiving countries, and consequences for family before deportation decisions are made (Human Rights Watch, 2009). In fact, most other major democracies around the world consider family relationships and other ties to the country before making deportation determinations (Human Rights Watch, 2007). The loss of judicial discretion in American removal proceedings, coupled with the expansion of non-violent triggering offenses, has greatly increased opportunities for family separation while obscuring the system's ostensible purpose of ensuring community safety and national security.

Meanwhile, noncitizens who commit crimes that are not aggravated felonies also face reduced opportunities for relief. Instead of having to show that their removal would cause "extreme hardship" to themselves or to a spouse, parent, or child—as they did under previous law—they now must show that their removal would cause "exceptional and extremely unusual hardship" (National Immigration Law Center, 2001, p. 7). This standard for "cancellation of removal" is so difficult to meet that approvals have averaged only 1,268 annually, despite the fact that the government is permitted to grant up to 4,000 petitions each year (Feinstein, 2004, p. 2). While no court has questioned the validity of the standard itself, the right to present evidence in support of an application for cancellation of removal has been confirmed. In *Cardenas-Morfin v. Ashcroft* (2004), the Ninth Circuit Court of Appeals found that an immigration judge violated an immigrant's due process rights when she precluded him from testifying about the hardship his 2-year old daughter would suffer if separated from her father.

IMPACT ON FAMILY INTEGRITY

According to the Pew Hispanic Center (Passel & Cohn, 2009), the number of United States-born children with unauthorized immigrant parents (children in "mixed status" families) grew from 2.7 million in 2003 to 4 million in 2008. Of all children with undocumented immigrant parents, 73% are born in the United States. Children with parents from Mexico and Central America are especially likely to live in mixed-status families (Fortuny, Capps, Simms & Chaudry, 2009), as are younger children. Of those younger than age 6 years whose parents are undocumented immigrants, 91% are born in the United States (Passel & Cohn, 2009). Because undocumented immigrants are by far the most likely to face deportation (Human Rights Watch, 2009) and such a large number (3.8 million) of them have citizen children, they are at the greatest risk for family separation.

Undocumented immigrants also have the fewest resources with which to navigate the immigration system. As a group, they are far less educated than residents born in the United States, with 47% of those between ages 25 and 64 years having less than a high school education. In 2007, their median household income was $36,000, considerably less than that of residents born in the United States. This disparity is even more striking since household sizes in these families tend to be larger, and incomes are less likely to rise in accordance with time spent in the United States. Not surprisingly, unauthorized immigrants are more likely than American-born residents to live in poverty and less likely to have health insurance (Passel & Cohn, 2009).

Despite the gravity of what is at stake in immigration trials (loss of home, work, family, and community), they are considered to be "civil" rather than "criminal" proceedings. As such, the government is under no obligation to provide free legal representation. In 2006, only 35% of the 113,140 individuals appearing in immigration court were represented (Schoenholtz & Bernstein, 2008); in some areas of the country, as few as 10% of detainees have counsel (Families for Freedom, n.d.). Not surprisingly, immigrants without legal representation are far less successful than those who have representation. For example, in fiscal year 2003, 34% of non-detained immigrants with attorneys won their cases compared to 23% without. Among those seeking asylum, 39% with attorneys won their cases, compared to 14% of those without (Ferguson, 2007). Immigration law is highly complex. Imagine how daunting it is for those with little education or income and few basic English skills. Whatever claims for relief may exist (premised on refugee status, domestic violence, human trafficking, or being a victim of a serious crime), the chances for success are greatly diminished absent legal representation. The consequences can be, and often are, devastating for families.

The Department of Homeland Security estimates that of the 2,199,138 removals conducted between fiscal years 1998 and 2007, 108,434 involved parents of American-citizen children. If multiple removals of the same parent are included (those who are deported, return, and are deported again), the number increases by an additional 72,000 (Office of Inspector General, 2009). No data, however, are available on how many children are affected or on what becomes of those who are left behind. Parents facing deportation confront a no-win proposition: they can rip their children, who have legal citizenship rights, from the only home they have known and return them to an alien land and uncertain future in order to keep the family intact, or they can relinquish their children to relatives or child welfare authorities in the United States and endure indefinite separation. Our immigration law forces parents into a "choiceless choice" (Thronson, 2006, p. 1211).

When parents sacrifice their children's constitutional right to remain in the United States for the sake of family integrity, the children suffer what some have termed *de facto* or "constructive" removal. Despite legal guarantees that prohibit the deportation of U.S. citizens, that is effectively what occurs for thousands of U.S.-born children each year. While these children may *possess* a right to remain in the country, they are not necessarily at liberty to *exercise* that right. Judges generally expect that children will remain with their parents if the parents are deported; yet the child's life chances—for education, safety, and freedom—may be better served by remaining in the United States. No parent should be forced to weigh their children's interest in remaining with family against the prospects for a better life, yet that is exactly what our immigration laws require. It is clear that "protecting children and their interests is not a priority of immigration law" (Thronson, 2006, p. 1180).

This holds equally true when parents facing deportation leave their citizen children behind. Not only are parents and children separated, but deportation may result in what some have termed *de facto* termination of parental rights. Under the Adoption and Safe Families Act of 1997, states must petition to terminate parental rights for any child who has been in out-of-home care for 12 of the most recent 22 months. Parents facing deportation, despite their best efforts, are highly unlikely to be able to reunify with their children within this timeframe. At best, they will have to return to their home countries and initiate the immigration process. At worst, they will be barred from reentry for 5 to 10 years (in the case of unauthorized immigrants) or permanently (in the case of aggravated felons). The outcome here flies in the face of family law's recognition of the sanctity of parent–child relationships. Ordinarily, termination of parental rights requires a finding that the parent is unfit. No such finding is present here. Furthermore, "in contrast to the safeguards provided to parents facing a termination of their parental rights, immigration removal hearings are largely devoid of such procedural safeguards" (Ferguson, 2007, p. 96). By deporting the parent, we may be subverting what is in the child's best interests and what drives our child welfare policy: safety, stability, and well-being. "A parent's immigration status or citizenship status per se is irrelevant to the determination of a child's best interests because it says absolutely nothing about the parenting of any person or rights of that person in the parent–child relationship" (Thronson, 2008, p. 466). By the same token, in two-parent households where one parent is deported, a *de facto* child custody determination can result. Again, the best interests of the child are irrelevant to the actual decision. Reflecting on a case in which an unauthorized immigrant was removed with his child, Thronson (2008) observes, "Whatever decision regarding child custody would have resulted from a family law proceeding is unknown because immigration law effectively resolved the issue without consideration of any of the factors that would have been relevant to a court determining the best interests of the child" (p. 510). Custody determinations are designed to be flexible; immigration proceedings are unyielding.

Whatever decision is made, there are enormous consequences for the child and for the integrity of the family:

> If a parent is deported, the action can initiate a child's entry into the foster care system. On the other hand, a child may accompany the deported parent while other family members remain in the United States, but then the family is separated. If the deported parent is the primary wage earner, the family members who remain in the United States may be catapulted into economic jeopardy. (Pine & Drachman, 2005, p. 549)

Unfortunately, legal challenges to the failure of immigration judges to consider family ties have been uniformly unsuccessful. In one notable case, however, a federal judge in Brooklyn ruled that immigration authorities must consider the potential impact on a child before deporting the child's parent (*Beharry v. Reno*, 2002). The case concerned a man from Trinidad who had entered the country at age 7 years as a legal permanent resident. Nineteen years later, still living in the United States, he was convicted of stealing $714 from a coffee shop. During his incarceration, passage of the 1996 immigration laws led to his designation as an aggravated felon. He was ultimately deported, leaving his U.S.-citizen daughter in the care of a grandmother. The District Court found that his removal violated the United Nations Convention on the Rights of the Child and the Universal Declaration of Human Rights since it failed to consider the best interests of the child. On appeal (*Beharry v. Ashcroft*, 2003), the decision was overturned on procedural grounds. Circuit Court Judge (now U.S. Supreme Court Justice) Sonia Sotomayor, writing for the court, never reached the merits of the "best interests" argument. Subsequent cases, however, have been unanimous in rejecting the proposition that a child's best interests must be considered as part of removal proceedings.

THE CHILD CITIZEN PROTECTION ACT OF 2009

Motivated largely by security fears and opposition to "illegal" immigration, the United States Congress has made repeated attempts to reform our immigration laws. Pressure for comprehensive reform during the 110th Congress led to the introduction of multiple bills and exhaustive negotiations around immigration enforcement, guest worker provisions, and a path to citizenship for undocumented residents. With pressure mounting from both the right and the left, a fragile coalition supporting the compromise measure in the Senate (S.1639) fell apart and the bill died after failing to survive a cloture vote to end debate. Lost in the shuffle was a modest bill introduced by Representative Jose Serrano (D-NY), entitled the Child Citizen Protection Act. Originally introduced in the 109th Congress, it would restore the ability of immigration judges to consider the best interests of the child in making removal determinations. The bill applies only to immigrant parents of citizen children and outlines exceptions for parents who pose a security threat or have engaged in human trafficking. As Representative Serrano explains,

> Currently, an immigration judge presiding over cases that would separate parents from children, has no choice but to order permanent removal of the undocumented parent from the United States. There is no room to consider the harm such separation would cause to the child, who is a citizen. As a result of this, the parents who do have citizenship have been forced to become single parents, dependents have become breadwinners, and working American families have joined the welfare rolls. Most importantly, the children, who bear no blame, have lost contact with a parent and intact families are broken apart. The present immigration system does little to protect the best interests of the children and keep families together ... Children deserve better than to lose a parent because of an inflexible law. (2006, p. 1)

The bill was reintroduced in the current Congress as H.R. 182. Two primary arguments have been lodged against it. Some maintain that parents who face separation from their children due to deportation have only themselves to blame; they should have considered the consequences before acting illegally. Others believe that allowing parents to avoid deportation because they have U.S.-born "anchor babies" will only encourage illegal immigration. Both arguments miss the point. A society that purports to value family should exercise every reasonable opportunity to keep parents and children together—especially when, as under current law, parents can be deported for a whole host of reasons that have little to do with domestic security and may well be outweighed by the best interests of their children.

Many mainstream immigration rights groups agree with the bill in principle, but have been hesitant to throw their weight behind it because they perceive it as being too radical in the current, anti-immigrant climate. The most visible support comes from a grassroots organization in New York called Families for Freedom. Together with Representative Serrano's office, they have used the bill to educate the public about who "illegal" immigrants really are and what "criminal" really means in the immigration context. In this way, they hope to alter the terms of the debate. Another organization, American Fraternity, has taken a different approach. Using many of the same arguments that underlie the Child Citizen Protection Act, they sought (unsuccessfully) to file a class action lawsuit to halt the deportation of undocumented parents with citizen children (*Sandigo v. Obama*, 2009). These and other groups have organized rallies, town hall meetings, and vigils to sensitize the public and politicians to the plight of citizen children with noncitizen parents.

Meanwhile, preparation for another round of immigration reform continues on Capitol Hill. On December 15, 2009, Representative Solomon Ortiz (D-TX) introduced the Comprehensive Immigration Reform for America's Security and Prosperity Act (CIR ASAP, H.R. 4321). Tucked into this 645-page bill, as one small provision, is the text of the Child Citizen Protection Act. The Comprehensive Immigration Reform bill has 102 co-sponsors to date and the support of the Congressional Hispanic Caucus whose Immigration Task Force is chaired by Representative Luis Gutierrez (D-IL), a social worker. It was referred to nine different Congressional committees and is expected to move forward as *the* House immigration bill when Congress takes up the issue later this year.

ALTERNATIVE REMEDIES

While inclusion of the Child Citizen Protection Act in the larger immigration reform bill provides it with some political cover, its future remains uncertain. It is therefore important to pursue other strategies to reduce the number of families separated through deportation. Providing indigent parents facing removal with free legal counsel should be a high priority. "Many times individuals slated for removal hearings have difficulty procuring representation because they do not know how to go about finding counsel, do not have the resources to pay a private-sector lawyer, and/or are detained and thus even more limited in their information about and access to counsel" (Schoenholtz & Bernstein, 2008). The American Bar Association adopted a resolution in 2006, supporting "the due process right to counsel for all persons in removal proceedings, and the availability of legal representation to all non-citizens in immigration-related matters" (Pena, 2006, p. 1). Most states already provide low-income parents with lawyers when child custody or termination of parental rights is at issue. As we observed earlier, deportation proceedings that threaten to separate parents from their citizen children can be tantamount to child custody determinations or *de facto* terminations of parental rights. If counsel is necessary to ensure due process in these family court proceedings, it should be considered equally indispensible in federal immigration cases. A guarantee of representation by counsel could assist thousands of parents in understanding and navigating the complexities of the immigration system, thereby maximizing the likelihood of positive outcomes for them and their children.

Another remedy would be to roll back some of the changes instituted under the 1996 immigration and welfare reform laws. These laws pander to the public's anxiety about immigration and move us away from rationally addressing the legitimate goals of immigration policy. The current definition of what constitutes a deportable "aggravated felony" should be repealed in favor of a narrower definition that targets violent crime. Representative Bob Filner (D-CA) has introduced a bill (H.R. 938) to that effect. Similarly, the provision that requires a showing of "exceptional and extremely unusual hardship" for cancellation of removal should be repealed in favor of one that permits consideration of deportation's potentially devastating consequences for families with children. Meanwhile, access to federal benefit programs curtailed by the 1996 welfare reform bill should be restored; in the event that one family member is deported, remaining family members would have the resources they need to keep the family intact.

Reducing the number of deportations within families could also be achieved by limiting the role of local law enforcement in apprehending and reporting undocumented immigrants. Under agreements authorized by Section 287(g) of the Immigration and Nationality Act, state and local law enforcement officials can partner with ICE to enforce federal immigration laws. Between 2006 and 2009, more than 120,000 undocumented immigrants were identified for removal as a result of 287(g) agreements in 77 jurisdictions across 25 states (Feere, 2009). Data confirm that most of these immigrants are held on alcohol-related charges or for possession of fake identification (Green & Walker, 2007), not for violent crimes. Law enforcement professionals in many jurisdictions—including Arizona, which recently passed the nation's harshest anti-immigration law—oppose participation in 287(g) agreements; they fear that the program will jeopardize community safety by dissuading victims and witnesses from cooperating with police. Speaking out at the local level against implementation of these partnerships could result in fewer immigrants being detained and deported for minor offenses.

There is no question that family integrity is best protected by preventing unnecessary detentions and removals. Much can be done in the meantime, however, to mitigate the effects of family separation when it does occur. The Comprehensive Immigration Reform bill referenced earlier contains numerous provisions that aim to do just that. Many of these provisions address government raids at work sites and private homes. Some center on ensuring access to information about legal counsel, while others are designed to facilitate the involvement of state or local service agencies "including relevant nongovernmental organizations, child welfare agencies, child protective service agencies, school and head start administrators, mental health and legal service providers, and hospitals" (H.R. 4321, Sec. 151(8)). Families with children are afforded special protections in relation to both apprehension and detention, including an:

- opportunity for parents to arrange for the care of dependent children;
- confidential psychosocial and mental health services;
- free legal advice about child welfare and custody determinations;
- contact information for child welfare service providers; and
- access to communication with extended family members.

Steps are also required to minimize the trauma experienced by children including avoiding apprehensions, interrogations and screenings in the child's presence. Other provisions make special accommodations for vulnerable populations including women who are pregnant or nursing; children; parents detained with one or more of their children; those who provide financial, physical, and other direct support to minor children, parents, or other dependents; people with disabilities, older adults, and victims of abuse (H.R. 4321, Sec. 160). The bill would generally prohibit families with children from being separated or taken into custody except in limited circumstances, and would require that those who are detained be placed in "non-penal, residential, home-like facilities that enable families to live as a family" and that are managed by staff with demonstrated expertise in child welfare (H.R. 4321, Sec. 162(c)(2)). Finally, the bill would require various memoranda of understanding and collaborations among the Department of Homeland Security, the Department of Health and Human Services, state and local child welfare agencies, law enforcement, and local mental health professionals, including mandatory joint training and the development of joint protocols that prioritize the best interests of the child and family (H.R. 4321, Sec. 164-167).

IMPLICATIONS FOR CHILD WELFARE

When immigration law fails to consider the best interests of the child, family integrity is compromised. Child welfare agencies can play a role in minimizing the resulting harm—both with families already in the system, and with families that are impacted by immigration enforcement. Child welfare staff should be knowledgeable not only about the many practice issues that arise with immigrant families, but also about the policies that affect their well-being. The legal interactions between the immigration and child welfare systems are complex; consulting with immigration attorneys, or developing in-house expertise on immigration matters, can help workers avoid inadvertent missteps that might jeopardize a child or family's future.

When families are already involved with the child welfare system, ascertaining the immigration status of each family member (including nuclear family, extended family, and fictive kin) is a crucial starting point. It enables the agency to work with the family to develop a plan around who should provide short-term, emergency care for the children if a noncitizen parent is apprehended. It can also help the agency identify who might qualify to serve as a foster parent, adoptive parent, or legal guardian if a parent is deported. Agency staff should familiarize themselves with state policies defining eligibility to serve in these capacities. In Texas, for example, only citizens and legal permanent residents can be foster or adoptive parents; however, the Director of Child Welfare has the authority to grant a waiver if it is in the child's best interests (Texas Department of Family and Protective Services, n.d.). Having a plan in place to address unexpected separations can minimize confusion and help insure child safety. It can make the transition as seamless as possible by increasing the chances of placement with relatives, friends, or trusted members of the family's own community.

Implementing such a plan may require extraordinary efforts on the agency's part to locate and engage family members who can assume responsibility for separated children. A number of states have had success using family group conferencing for this purpose. In situations where extended family members reside both in the United States and in a foreign country, cross-border family group conferencing can be initiated. The goal is to "involve, engage, and encourage permanent connections with the broadest family constellations" (Howard & Bruce, 2008, p. 1). This goal can be facilitated by collaborations with foreign consulates, social service agencies, and non-governmental organizations. A number of border towns have established international liaison offices within their departments of health and human services. In San Diego and El Paso, for example, "in addition to helping search for parents and relatives, the liaison office helps complete background checks and home studies, and assists with visitation, placement, and services across borders" (Howard & Bruce, 2008, p. 3).

To do justice to immigrant families involved with the child welfare system, agency social workers should also be familiar with the various circumstances under which noncitizen family members might be eligible for immigration relief. For example, special consideration is available for victims of human trafficking (asylum, T-Visa), victims of abuse (Violence Against Women Act [VAWA]), and victims of serious crime (U-Visa). If parents are successful in adjusting their immigration status and moving toward citizenship, family stability is enhanced. Consulting with an immigration attorney is critical in these instances since making an application can be risky; it can place the applicant's noncitizen status on Homeland Security's radar, thus rendering the parent even more vulnerable to detection and removal.

Determining a family's immigration status, while important, is not always easy. Parents may be confused about their immigration status, particularly in mixed-status families. Children may be misinformed and language barriers may make accurate communication difficult. Finally, concerns about deportation may make families hesitant to disclose their status; to many, child welfare workers and immigration officials are indistinguishable. For this reason, some recommend using proxy questions including country of origin, language spoken at home, or length of time in the United States (New Mexico Children's Law Center, n.d.), rather than asking clients directly about their status. It is likewise advisable to partner with grass-roots organizations that have already developed trusting relationships with a particular immigrant community. In any case, workers should assure their clients that the information will be kept confidential. They must also be clear about their obligation as service providers to safeguard their clients' rights. Unfortunately, some professionals—including police, probation officers, juvenile detention staff, prosecutors, public defenders, judges, eligibility workers, and child welfare staff—may mistakenly believe they have a legal duty to report undocumented immigrant parents and children to ICE. In 2009, a social worker under contract with the Florida Department of Children and Families turned in an undocumented Guatemalan mother while she was visiting with her two U.S. citizen children. A week later, that same social worker arranged a visit between the children and their Guatemalan grandparents so that local authorities could apprehend them as well (Florida Immigrant Coalition, 2009). Having information about a client's immigration status should trigger the ethical obligation to use it only in ways that promote the child's best interests. Immigration laws explicitly preserve the right to legally access child welfare services, regardless of one's immigration status.

There are other ways in which social workers' biases can jeopardize a child's best interests. Working with foreign countries to resolve placement issues can tax one's professional objectivity and cultural humility. It requires child welfare staff to weigh "the benefits and opportunities for children that may be available in the United States against the loss of culture, language, family traditions, values, and beliefs that each family holds" (Howard & Bruce, 2008, p. 4). In addition, agencies must guard against using a family's immigration status as a reason to deny services or to avoid pursuing kinship placements. Assumptions that such placements would necessarily be unstable are erroneous; the fact "that undocumented immigrants are here without authorization does not necessarily mean that their deportation is imminent" (Morrison & Thronson, 2010, p. 6). Given the unique challenges faced by children in immigrant families, the benefits of kinship care may be especially important. Finally, determinations of parental fitness should never be premised on immigration status. Recently, the Supreme Court of Nebraska considered the case of a Guatemalan mother with four children whose parental rights had been terminated (*In re Interest of Angelica L.*,

2009). In reversing the termination decision, the court found that the state had failed to provide clear and convincing evidence of the mother's unfitness as a parent, relying instead on the fact of her arrest and deportation.

In addition to tending to their own clients, social workers have been instrumental in addressing the needs of other children who become entangled in immigration enforcement activities. In Massachusetts, for example, child welfare workers served as first responders following a mass work site raid in New Bedford. It was the child welfare workers who offered support to detainees and took responsibility for children who were abandoned and traumatized by the sudden disappearance of their parents. They worked to obtain the release of adults who were primary caretakers of underage children and aided parents in planning for the possibility of deportation (Capps et al., 2007). These are functions that public child welfare agencies can implement even in the absence of changes to federal law. Relationships with community-based immigration organizations should be forged now, and plans for a coordinated a response developed, so that help can be mobilized on short notice whenever the need arises.

While child welfare professionals continue to care for children who are separated from their parents, they must also be vigilant in pressing for policy changes that will minimize the number of deportations. This vigilance includes seeking to limit the number of 287(g) agreements between local law enforcement and ICE, pressuring the Obama administration to limit enforcement activities and to ensure that they are conducted in a manner that respects the special needs of children, and generating public support for rolling back the draconian changes instituted in the 1996 immigration and welfare reform laws. As Congress again considers comprehensive immigration reform, potential impacts on children must be kept front and center; legislators need to understand the dilemmas confronting mixed status families and be convinced that stable, intact families of all kinds make our nation stronger. Finally, whatever its prospects, we must persist in supporting the principles behind the Child Citizen Protection Act. An immigration system that ignores the best interests of the child is unacceptable.

CONCLUSION

Approximately four million U.S. citizen children are currently living in mixed-status families. More than 100,000 parents in these families have been deported over the past 10 years. Immigration enforcement has been accelerated at the local, state, and national levels and current policies make removal easier and exceptions fewer. U.S. citizen children with noncitizen parents continue to be burdened by the intolerable prospect of family separation. Meanwhile, critical information is lacking, creating important opportunities for research. When faced with deportation, how many children leave the country with their parents? How many remain in the United States? What becomes of those children who remain in this country? Anecdotal evidence suggests that some are cared for by relatives while others enter foster care. Unless we actively engage in advocating for proposals that protect family integrity, such as the Child Citizen Protection Act, we are destined to see more traumatized children come through our doors—victims of America's misguided immigration laws. "Immigration policy must respect the importance of human relationships. No policy should result in family separation" (Padilla, Shapiro, Fernandez-Castro & Faulkner, 2008, p. 6).

The truth is that much of our immigration policy is at odds with the goals of child welfare. Rather than promote children's safety, stability, and well-being, "immigration law results in decisions about children that are not motivated in the least by consideration of the children's best interests" (Thronson, 2008, p. 511). Conflicting policies have created a perverse situation in which "family integrity can be maintained only by violating the nation's immigration laws and vice versa" (Ferguson, 2007, p. 87). Child welfare advocates have been passionate and effective in pressing for improved child welfare laws. We need to remain equally passionate in challenging policies in other spheres that impact vulnerable children. With comprehensive immigration reform again on the national horizon, opportunities abound. Meanwhile, there is much that child welfare agencies can do here and now, including assisting eligible families in regularizing their status, preparing families for the possibility of separation, and identifying kin and fictive kin who might qualify as temporary or permanent caregivers. Child welfare professionals can also play a leadership role in assisting families and children displaced by immigration enforcement activities. Finally, it is essential to forge new partnerships: with grass-roots organizations in immigrant communities, with foreign embassies and social service agencies, with local law enforcement, and with immigration attorneys. The U.S. child welfare system needs to broaden its horizons by assuming nontraditional roles and engaging in new collaborative relationships. In this way, the system can successfully promote family integrity and ensure that children in immigrant families achieve the safety, stability, and well-being they deserve.

REFERENCES

Adoption and Safe Families Act (1997), P.L. 104–132.
Adoption Assistance and Child Welfare Act (1980), P.L. 96–272.
Antiterrorism and Effective Death Penalty Act (1996), P.L. 104–132.
Beharry v. Ashcroft, 329 F.2d 51 (2nd Cir. 2003).
Beharry v. Reno, 1832 F.Supp.2d 588 (2002).
Borelli, K., Earner, I., & Lincroft, Y. (2007). Administrators in public child welfare: Responding to immigrant families. *Protecting Children, 22*(2), 8–19.
Capps, R. (2008). *Five questions for Randy Capps*. Washington, DC: Urban Institute.

Capps, R., Castenada, R. M., Chaudry, A., & Santos, R. (2007). *Paying the price: The impact of immigration raids on America's children*. Washington, DC: National Council of La Raza.

Cardenas–Morfin v. Ashcroft, 87 Fed. Appx. 629 (2004).

Dettlaff, A., & Phillips, S. D. (2007, November). *Immigration enforcement considerations for child welfare systems*. Chicago, IL: Jane Addams College of Social Work.

Families for Freedom. (n.d.). *About us*. Retrieved from http://www.familiesforfreedom.org/httpdocs/about_us.html

Family Preservation and Support Services Program Act (1993), P.L. 103–66.

Feere, J. (2009). *The Obama administration's 287(g): An analysis of the new MOA*. Center for Immigration Studies. Retrieved from http://www.cis.org/ObamasNew287g

Feinstein, D. (2004, June 4). *Senator Feinstein questions deportation of long–term, law–abiding undocumented immigrants*. Retrieved from http://feinstein-senate.gov/04Releases/r–hutchison–ltr–removal.htm

Ferguson, S. A. (2007). Not without my daughter: Deportation and the termination of parental rights. *Georgetown Immigration Law Journal, 22*, 85–104.

Florida Immigrant Coalition (2009). *Overzealous immigration enforcement hurts and angers community members*. Media Alert. Retrieved from www.floridaimmigrant.org

Fortuny, K., Capps, R., Simms, M., & Chaudry, A. (2009). *Children of immigrants: National and state characteristics*. Washington, DC: Urban Institute.

Illegal Immigration Reform and Immigrant Responsibility Act (1996), P.L. 104–208.

Green, F., & Walker, K. (2007, August 31). *Manassas Journal Messenger*, p. A1.

Howard, M., & Bruce, L. (2008). Using family group conferencing to assist immigrant children and families in the child welfare system. Retrieved from American Humane Association website: http://www.americanhumane.org/assets/docs/protecting–children/PC–fgdm–immigrant–children–families.pdf

Human Rights Watch (2007). *Forced apart: Families separated and immigrants harmed by United States deportation policy*. New York, NY: Author.

Human Rights Watch (2009). *Forced apart (by the numbers): Non–citizens deported mostly for nonviolent offenses*. New York, NY: Author.

Immigration and Nationality Act (1952), P.L. 82–414.

Immigration and Nationality Act (1965), P.L. 89–236.

In re Interest of Angelica L., 767 N.W.2d 74 (2009).

Kremer, J. D., Moccio, K. A., & Hammell, J. W. (2009). *Severing a lifeline: The neglect of citizen children in America's immigration enforcement policy*. Retrieved from http://www.dorsey.com/files/upload/DorseyProBono_SeveringLifeline_web.pdf

McKay, R. (2003). *Family reunification*. Retrieved from http://www.migrationinformation.org/USFocus/print.cfm?ID–122

Monger, R., & Rytina, N. (2009). *Annual flow report: U.S. legal permanent residents: 2008*. Washington, DC: United States Department of Homeland Security.

Morrison, A. D., & Thronson, D. B. (2010). Beyond status: Seeing the whole child. *Evaluation and Program Planning, 33*, 281–287.

National Immigration Law Center. (2001). BIA issues decisions interpreting standards in suspension and cancellation cases. *Immigrants' Rights Update, 15*(4), 7–8.

New Mexico Children's Law Center. (n.d.). *Child protection best practices bulletin: Working with undocumented and mixed status immigrant children and families.* Retrieved from http://ipl.unm.edu/childlaw/pub,php

Office of Inspector General (2009). *Removals involving illegal alien parents of United States citizen children.* Washington, DC: United States Department of Homeland Security.

Padilla, Y. C., Shapiro, E. R., Fernandez-Castro, M. D., & Faulkner, M. (2008). Our nation's immigrants in peril: An urgent call to social workers. *Social Work, 53*(1), 5–8.

Passel, J. S., & Cohn, D. (2009). *A portrait of unauthorized immigrants in the United States.* Washington, DC: Pew Hispanic Center.

Pena, R. (2006). *The quest to fulfill our nation's promise of liberty and justice for all: ABA policies on issues affecting immigrants and refugees.* Washington, DC: American Bar Association Commission on Immigration.

Personal Responsibility and Work Opportunity Reconciliation Act (1996), P.L. 104–193.

Pine, B. A., & Drachman, D. (2005). Effective child welfare practice with immigrant and refugee children and their families. *Child Welfare, 84*, 537–562.

Rome, S. H. (2008). Untangling the web: Immigration law and child welfare practice. *Michigan Child Welfare Law Journal, 12*(1), 14–22.

Sandigo v. Obama (2009), U.S. Dist. LEXIS 110684.

Schoenholtz, A., & Bernstein, H. (2008). Improving immigration adjudications through competent counsel. *Georgetown Journal of Legal Ethics, 21*(1), 55–60.

Serrano, J. E. (2006, March 29). *Serrano introduces "Child Citizen Protection Act"* [press release]. Retrieved from http://Serrano.house.gov/Newsdetail.aspx?ID=207

Texas Department of Family and Protective Services (n.d.). *Inquiry and screening of foster family homes and adoptive homes.* CPS Handbook. Retrieved from http://www.dfps.state.tx.us/handbooks/CPS/Files/CPS_pg_7120.jsp

Thronson, D. B. (2006, Spring). Choiceless choices: Deportation and the parent–child relationship. *Nevada Law Journal, 6*, 1165–1214.

Thronson, D. B. (2008, February). Custody and contradictions: Exploring immigration law as federal family law in the context of child custody. *Hastings Law Journal, 59*, 453–513.

United States Immigration and Customs Enforcement (2007). *FY07 accomplishments.* Retrieved from www.ice.gov

Learning How to Dance with the Public Child Welfare System: Mexican Parents' Efforts to Exercise Their Voice

CECILIA AYÓN, EUGENE AISENBERG and PAULINE ERERA

The purpose of this article is to understand how Mexican parents' perceive their voices (their concerns, dissatisfaction, and opinions) as integrated in child welfare cases and what factors hinder or promote this process. The focus is on parents' interactions with their child welfare worker during routine monthly home visits. Nineteen parents, with a history of immigration, participated in in-depth interviews for this qualitative study. Grounded theory methods were used to complete the content analysis. The findings indicate that there are three principal factors that affect parents' decisions to exercise their voice: 1) parent's perceptions of how workers received their voice; 2) case context, including immigration status and fear of loosing children; and 3) the lack of parental knowledge and understanding of the child welfare case process and support/advocacy agents. Recommendations include utilizing empowerment models and culturally grounded practices that facilitate the integration of parents' voices in the parent–worker interactions and case process, and continued support for peer support interventions and formal forms of advocacy.

[The child welfare workers] were saying there were fractures on the leg and I was 100% sure that I didn't do it ... it's kind of hard you know when you are sure that you didn't do it ... there isn't much you can say ... If they would have believed us—that it wasn't us—then they wouldn't have taken the baby away from us. They didn't believe us ...

We went to court and [my husband] found out that [our daughter] was going to go for adoption and that's when he said no we are leaving, they are taking her from us ... I just started packing everything and we put everything in the car ... We took our daughter ... She was in foster care, we kidnapped our daughter and took her to Mexico. When we came back my husband got arrested ... he went to jail and they started looking for me and my daughter. So I had to turn her in ... [because] they were still going to take her away ...

She was receiving special treatment and she went to different doctors ... they found out that she had brittle bones. It's called osteogenesis imperfecta ... that made everything [better] for us, but everything that we had already been through was already there.

—Mrs. Gomez, a mother with an open child welfare case

Parent engagement and participation in involuntary child welfare cases is a growing area of interest to scholars and practitioners (Brown, 2006; Dumbrill, 2006). When families are dissatisfied with services, they do not have the option of exiting or discontinuing services (such is the case for child welfare cases); thus, exercising their voice is the only option they have to express their dissatisfaction, concerns, or thoughts (Hirschman, 1970). The families involved with the public child welfare system are highly stigmatized and isolated throughout the case process. Parents often feel powerless, controlled, and may lack the knowledge to navigate complex service systems, such as the child welfare system (Kemp, Marcenko, Hoagwook, & Vesneski, 2009; Frame, Conley, & Berrick, 2006). Among Latino families less is known about how parents negotiate exercising their voice (i.e., voicing their opinions, concerns, and feelings about the case) and how parents' perceive workers' reactions to their voice. As for most families, entering the public child welfare system can be an overwhelming experience for Latino families, in particular for those with a recent history of immigration, because this may be their first interaction with a large and unfamiliar bureaucratic system.

Promoting families' strengths and empowerment process is core to social work practice and should be a key component in child welfare interventions as the aim is to create a change that will protect and promote children's well-being. When parents' voices are excluded, they are not being actively engaged in the case process—an experience that can have significant implications in their families' lives (e.g., ranging from children's permanent removal to positive changes that promote family well-being such as recovery from substance abuse). Also, minimizing or discounting the voice of Latino families and their wisdom, values, needs, and experiences significantly hinders the utilization and provision of culturally competent services.

Engaging Latino parents in culturally responsive ways is vital as evidence highlights that Latino children and their families experience differential outcomes in the child welfare system. For example, compared with White children, Latino children tend to be younger at the referral and substantiation stage (Alzate & Rosenthal, 2009; Church, Gross, & Baldwin, 2005), are placed in out of home placements or enter state custody more quickly (Church et al., 2005), and spend a significantly longer period of time in foster care (Church, 2006). Even when White children in foster care report fewer symptoms of mental health problems, they are more likely than Latino children to receive needed and appropriate mental health services (Garland, Landsverk, & Lau, 2003). Neglecting to engage Latino children and families with respect or understanding of their histories, traditions, and value systems may contribute to these disparities.

The purpose of this article is to examine how Mexican parents who have an open case with the public child welfare system describe the extent to which their voices are incorporated in their case process and what factors contribute to or hinder such incorporation. This article focuses on Mexican families with a recent history of immigration (first and second generation) because there is much heterogeneity by Latino subgroups, specifically in regard to immigration generation. This article is guided by the following questions: What hinders parents from exercising their voice? When do parents exercise their voice? How do parents' perceive their voice is received by their worker? The contribution of this article lies in its analysis of Latino immigrant parents' experience in exercising their voice with their case worker because this is not a well studied population within child welfare research and rarely is their experience of the client–worker relationship examined.

ENGAGING FAMILIES IN THE PUBLIC CHILD WELFARE SYSTEM

Studies aiming to examine parent engagement in cases with the public child welfare system have primarily focused on the parent–worker relationship (deBoer & Coady, 2007; Lee & Ayón, 2004) and satisfaction with services rendered (Kapp & Vela, 2004; Lee & Ayón, 2004). These studies have generally found positive results related to worker competencies, the role of the relationship in the case, and/or parents' satisfaction with services.

A closer look at the process and context of engagement reveals that parents are unaware of their rights when involved with the public child welfare system (Kapp & Propp, 2002). Also, families' case contexts were often characterized by the presence of pervasive negative feelings (Yatchmenoff, 2005) due to parents' mistrust of workers and the child welfare system. Parents' perception of how the worker (mis)uses power significantly impacted how parents negotiate interactions with the public child welfare system (Dumbrill, 2006).

Dumbrill (2006) examined how parents experience and negotiate child protection intervention and found that parents described their worker as exercising their power over the family or to support the family. Depending on how the worker used the power, the parent would either fight by openly challenging the worker; "play the game" by cooperating; or genuinely collaborate with the worker. Similarly, Brown (2006) identified that families often reported learning how to play the game; that is, learning what to say and do in order to have positive interactions with the worker. More often than not, workers and administrators measure families' engagement by the level of cooperation or compliance (Brown, 2006; Holland, 2000). As noted by Dawson and Berry (2002), "cooperative parents are less likely to face court proceedings or removal of their children," while "uncooperative parents may not be offered the services" they need (p. 294). By solely relying on cooperation as a measure of successful engagement, researchers and workers fail to capture whether families' needs are being met and parents' involvement in the decision-making process is curtailed (Corby, Millar, & Young, 1996). Consequently, workers and the public child welfare system often remain unaware of the families' potential contributions and assets to resolve issues at hand.

In light of child-centered policies such as the Adoption and Safe Families Act, many recent interventions have focused on family centered practices. Family centered practices aim to engage parents in service delivery leading to reunification (Alpert & Brinter, 2009). Such practices involve collaborative parent–worker relationships that are respectful, are strength based, and seek to break down power differentials (Petr & Entriken, 1995; Alpert & Brinter, 2009). One example is the Family Group Decision-Making (FGDM) model. FGDM was developed as a means of addressing the overrepresentation of Maori children in the New Zealand child welfare system and the institutional racism experienced by this community (American Humane Association, 2008). Family group decision-making brings together the family and extended family of the child in efforts to develop a plan for the care and protection in cases of confirmed child abuse or neglect (Crampton, 2006). FGDM meetings are initiated by child welfare agencies whenever a critical decision about a child is required (American Humane Association, 2008): "FGDM processes actively seek the collaboration and leadership of family groups in crafting and implementing plans that support the safety, permanency and well-being of their children" (p. 1). Other interventions that aim to facilitate parents' engagement include parent-to-parent role modeling (Cohen & Canan, 2006), foster parent-to-parent dyad relationships (Linares, Montalto, Li, & Oza, 2006), and mutual aid/support peer groups (Frame et al., 2006). These interventions have focused on developing informal sources of support, parent empowerment, and promoting parents learning from the experiences of other parents who have successfully negotiated the public child welfare system.

Although several efforts to engage parents in the case process are in place, disparate experiences continue among families serviced by the child welfare system. Many of the families who enter the public child welfare system tend to experience high levels of service needs and stressors related to poverty, substance abuse, and mental health (Dawson & Berry, 2002). Families' involvement with the public child welfare system has the potential to assist families in accessing needed services to address their multifaceted needs. Thus, engaging families is fundamental not only for the successful implementation of child welfare service plan but to future interactions with systems of care as families' experiences with the public child welfare system can potentially impact their help seeking behavior in the future (Diorio, 1992).

Barriers to Engaging Latino Families

In the past 10 years the number of Latino families entering the public child welfare system has nearly doubled (United States Department of Health and Human Services [US DHHS], 1997; 2007). Yet very little is known about their interactions with this institution. What is known is that Latino families and families of color are overrepresented in the child welfare system and disparate treatment of these ethnic minority families persist within this system (Hines, Lemon, Wyatt, & Merdinger, 2004). When Mexican families enter the public child welfare system, they are likely to encounter many barriers to feeling engaged by their worker because their parenting values may be questioned or misunderstood, they may have undocumented status, and their community may lack resources such as advocacy and financial support. Structural issues within the public child welfare system such as high case loads, limited time with workers, language barriers, and lack of cultural competency also compound the barriers faced by Mexican families. For example, whereas workers may be unaware of the special needs of this community (due to documentation status and lack of resources), families may also feel more vulnerable and afraid to challenge the worker's perceived (and actual) power.

The interactions of the Mexican population (and Latino population in general) with systems of care such as mental health services and child welfare services are highly stigmatized and often are not congruent with the cultural norms of this community (Snowden & Yamada, 2005). Being involved with the public child welfare system may be filled with shame for Mexican origin families as the well-being of the family unit is fundamental to their cultural values. When families become involved with the public child welfare system parents are informed that they do not "properly" care for their children. The public child welfare system identifies the reasons for families' involvement by a specifying a type of maltreatment to children (i.e., physical abuse, neglect). However, the family may be experiencing difficulties or extreme stressors related to poverty, or mental health needs (Hines et al., 2004). In addition, parenting practices may be misunderstood or misinterpreting by the worker due to cultural differences (Fontes, 2002). By labeling parents as unfit, the child welfare system challenges the core values of Mexican families and their parenting. This factor alone may impact how parents interact with their worker. However, at the same time because the family unit is fundamental to the Mexican community (Cauce & Domenech-Rodriguez, 2000) parents are likely to do everything in their power to ensure that their family is not fragmented.

Families with a recent history of immigration are likely to be fearful of their interactions with public systems, such as the child welfare system, as their documentation status may be questioned (Loue, Faust, & Bunce, 2000) and deportation take place. Concomitantly, families who have limited English language skills or who are monolingual Spanish speakers may also experience barriers if proficient bilingual and bicultural service providers are not available (Suleiman Gonzalez, 2004). If parents are unable to communicate with service providers or engage in relationships that are grounded in their value base they may be unable to trust their worker to share their needs and information and the worker is less able to be responsive to the family.

THEORETICAL FRAMEWORK

This study is informed by the strengths and empowerment perspectives. Mexican families have multiple strengths grounded in their cultural values. Although Mexican families encounter considerable barriers and injustices they are a resilient community. For example, their familial relations and extended kinship networks are a source of support when confronted with social injustices and their adaptation process to the United States (Baca Zinn, 1994). Empowerment models aim to bring about the voices (e.g., needs, opinions) of communities and enhance the ability of families to develop the power to act on their behalf in society (Gutiérrez, Parson, & Cox, 2003). The empowerment perspective characterizes the client-worker relationship as one of shared power, families and workers are viewed as resources, and dialogue and critical analysis is a core aspect of the relationship (Gutiérrez et al., 2003).

METHODS

Sampling Procedures

Purposive sampling was used to obtain a convenience sample of 19 parents with open child welfare cases. Following human subjects approval, parents were recruited in the waiting room of a child welfare agency in Southern California (referred to as "the department" in this article). Parents were approached by the researcher and informed about the study. Parents who were of Mexican origin, first or second generation in the United States, and who were involved with the department due to neglect and/or physical abuse were eligible (and invited) to participate. Recruitment was limited to those individuals who came to the department to see their child(ren), sign paper work, or pick up information/resources. As many services are home-based many parents were excluded from participating in the study. If parents elected to participate in an interview, an appointment was made to complete the interview.

Participants

Sixteen mothers and three fathers, representing 16 families, participated in in-depth semi-structured interviews. The number of children in each family ranged from one to six, and 21% ($n = 4$) of parents reported that they had twins. In terms of birthplace, 52% ($n = 10$) of parents were immigrants from Mexico and the remaining parents were born in the United States and children of Mexican immigrants. Parents' educational level ranged from sixth grade to some college or trade.

The 19 parents had current open cases with the public child welfare system as a result of alleged maltreatment to their child(ren). At the time of the interviews, parents had their case open between 2 months and 2 years. Of the 16 families, nine (or 56%) reported that their children had been in an out-of-home placement; 25% ($n = 4$) reported a child in foster care, 12.5% ($n = 2$) reported a child placed with relatives, and 12.5% ($n = 2$) reported children in both relative and foster placement. In 19% of the cases ($n = 3$), children had been returned to their families.

The reasons for being involved with the department were described as actual situations (i.e., drug abuse, domestic violence, dispute with children) whereas the department would categorize the case as physical abuse or neglect. This lack of concordance is an important distinction and can funda-mentally influence the dynamics of communication and interaction between the family and worker. The services mandated by the department may be child centered while the parent views the issues as a parent or family issue. Furthermore, parents define their needs in a more contextual manner than is currently done by the child welfare system (Lee & Ayón, 2007).

Interviews

In-depth semi-structured interviews were used to obtain parents' perceptions on their experiences in exercising their voice with the public child welfare system. The interview guide was designed by the author for this research. Sample questions include:

1) Did you have an opportunity to share your feelings about your case with your worker?
2) Did your worker ask you for your opinion on decisions that were made in your case?
3a) Were there times when you did not agree with something in your case?
3b) Did you have the opportunity to disagree with the caseworker?
3c) How did your case worker respond?

All questions were followed with the question, "Can you give me an example?" and other probing questions. The interview guide also included questions about the demographic information on the family, worker, and case, and the family's immigration history. The interviews were audiotaped with consent and completed in Spanish or English. Interviews ranged from 60 to 90 minutes in length. Interviews were conducted in the parents' home or at a local park, based on the participant's preference.

Content Analysis

This study utilized the procedures for content analysis outlined by Straus and Corbin (1990). This method was used as the aim of the study is to examine part of the case process (i.e., how parents' exercise voice). The content analysis was completed in two stages: open and axial coding. Throughout the analysis a constant comparative approach was used to compare incident to incident within and between interviews (Strauss & Corbin, 1990; Charmaz, 2006). Open coding involves four procedures: a) identifying and labeling each distinct incident or idea; b) categorizing the data by grouping concepts that represent similar phenomena; c) labeling or naming the categories; and d) developing properties and dimensions of the identified categories. The interviews were (re)read, labeled, and categorized.

In axial coding, connections between the categories and subcategories are made. Axial coding contextualizes the properties of the phenomenon by identifying the casual conditions by which the phenomenon is manifested and examining the consequences of the phenomena. In this study the axial coding focused on factors that hindered and promoted parents from exercising their voice, reasons parents exercised their voice, and the reception by the worker from the perspective of the parent. Moreover, axial coding involved constructing the model, linking the categories and subcategories, and describing the whole process (see Figure 1).

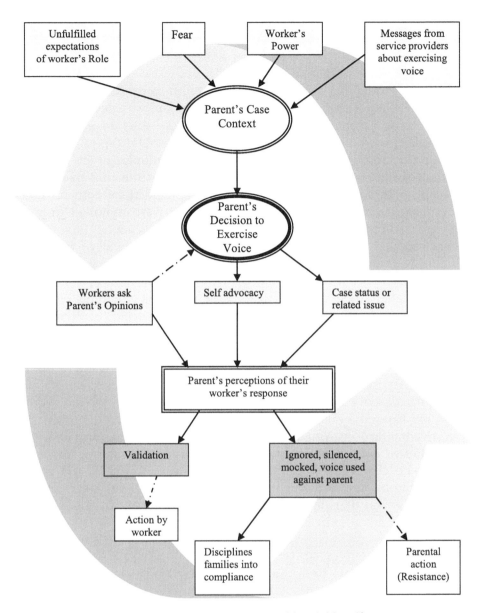

FIGURE 1 Parent's Voice in Ongoing Public Child Welfare Cases.

The lead author primarily completed the content analysis. All authors reviewed the model and interpretations. In case of a disagreement, the authors reviewed the transcripts. In the results section, parents' quotes are used extensively to support the model, thus addressing the validity and credibility of the model (Charmaz, 2005). For parents who elected to complete the interviews in Spanish, quotes are included with an English translation.

RESULTS AND DISCUSSION

Parents' Efforts to Exercise Their Voice

Figure 1 is a model that represents parents' effort to exercise their voice in ongoing child protection services cases. The model was developed based on the interview content and focuses on parents' interactions with their child welfare worker during monthly home visits. The typical child welfare trajectory requires families to interact with multiple service providers and child welfare workers. Thus, in this study, by the time parents are interacting with the worker, they had earlier interactions with an emergency response worker; in addition, if children were removed from the family, the parents also had interactions with a dependency investigator. Parents revealed several factors that influence the context of their case, including fear, worker's power, unfulfilled expectations of worker's role, and mixed messages from service providers. Also, they indicated that these factors also affect their decision to exercise their voice. Parents elected to exercise their voice to express service needs, to advocate for their family, and to ask questions or ask for information about their case, or when workers ask families for their opinions. Once parents exercised their voice, they felt they were either validated or ignored/silenced by their worker. In some cases, parents reported that their voice was used against them, the parents described being disciplined into compliance by the worker, or parents resisted by taking further action. Parents shared positive and supportive interactions with their worker; however, when parents expressed a complaint or need that the worker was unable to fulfill, the interaction tended to be characterized more negatively. As indicated by the circular arrows in the background, parents' effort to exercise their voice is an ongoing process and dynamic. The path experienced varies by the issue and parent.

What Hinders Parents From Exercising Their Voice or Speaking Out?

The context in which parents' cases are situated plays a significant role in their decision to exercise their voice. Note that the four factors (fear, worker's power, unfulfilled expectations of worker's role, and mixed messages from service providers) that influence the parent case context were not present from the very beginning (except for fear). Gradually parents learn about the worker's power, their expectations go unfulfilled, and from their interactions with other service providers they learn about the consequences to voicing their opinions. Moreover, families are not necessarily silent or compliant from the beginning.

Fear: Removal of Children and Immigration Status

Fear is at the core of parents' experiences and interactions with the child welfare system. Parents become vulnerable as they fear that their children can be removed or not returned. As noted by Diorio (1992) parents struggle to cope with overwhelming feelings of fear when faced with the possibility of losing their children. Mexican parents' connection to their children and family is fundamental to their well-being. A core value of the Mexican community, *familismo*, refers to the importance of family closeness/unity and getting along with and contributing to the well-being of the family (Cauce & Domenech-Rodriguez, 2000). The risk of the fragmentation of their family is likely to place the family members in a state of hyper-stress or as described by one mother "desde que empezó el caso yo estoy en un estado de nerviosismo que no se me ha quitado" ["since my case started I have been in a state of nervousness and it hasn't gone away"].

In addition, parents who were immigrants fear that their documentation status will play a role in their case or that being involved with the system will impact their chances of obtaining residency in the United States.

> *Uno de Hispano tiene mas miedo, mas temor, y mas uno de inmigrante, tiene mas miedo decir algo. Tengo 20 años yo de estar aquí seria una mentira decir que no ha aprendido muchas cosas ... de la vida Americana. Pero en realidad siento que es muy traumatisante pasar por esto. Yo no se lo deseo a nadie ... [No se] si me vaya afectar en mi record como que sea un cargo criminal. Como yo todavía no tengo mis papeles y estoy pensando en un futuro poder resolver mi situación legal en este país.*

> As a Hispanic one is more afraid, more frightened, even more if one is an immigrant, you are more afraid to say something. I've been here 20 years and it would be a lie if I said that I haven't learned a lot about the American life. But the truth is that I feel this is a very traumatic experience. I wouldn't wish this upon anyone. I don't know if this will affect my record like will this be a criminal crime. I still don't have my papers and in the future I would like to resolve my documentation situation in this country.

Parents' Perception of Workers' Power

Parents recognize the power that child welfare workers have to remove their children and to return their children. As workers have the power to make these crucial decisions (or influence the decision through their reports) parents often stated that it was very important to be liked by their worker. As one parent stated, "*Yo creo que si importa que le caiga bien a la trabajadora ... Es como la policía cuando abusa de la gente porque no le cae bien ...*

o es racista. Y puede pasar lo mismo con los trabajadores sociales" ["I think that it matters if the worker likes you ... It's like when a police man abuses people because he doesn't like them or because he is racist. The same could happen with the social workers"]. This quote also suggests that other factors are operative in the case. Parents' experience of racism as an ethnic minority and immigrant, in addition to their experiences with other systems, may also affect and inform their interactions with their worker. In the previous quote, it is noteworthy that the mother makes an association with police—those who wield power. Parents also stated that if the workers "did not like you", they are less likely to provide the support, guidance, or assistance needed to reunify families.

> When social workers don't like you it's harder. It's harder for you to do everything ... if you don't have [your kids] it matters a lot because it is up to the social worker for you to get more visitations, it is up to the social worker if she wants to help you get your kids back too. If I'm doing my part and the social worker is still saying no I don't think the kids should to go back with her, then that ... means that [the social worker] doesn't like me.

Parents' feared that if they were not liked by their worker they would be deemed uncooperative. Previous studies have confirmed that workers often assess families' progress based on their level of cooperation (Brown, 2006).

Unfulfilled Expectations of Workers' Role

Parents often described being confused about their worker's role. Parents revealed that workers present their role as someone who will provide assistance or "help" them get their children back. Parents expect the worker to be supportive and provide help in accessing information and/or advocating for them. For example, the following parent speaks to the power that the worker has and is upset that the worker does not use her position to advocate on the parent's behalf. This parent wants to increase the number of days that she sees her kids.

> I feel like [the worker] is using her authority when she wants ... she has power to make decisions. When we went to my mother in law's house to have that meeting she was pretty much asking my mother in law—is it ok if we increase the visits [from two times] to three times a week. Why does she need to ask her if she has the authority, she should be telling her, not asking her, and ... she told my mother-in-law over and over again that the purpose of the visits was to reunify the mother with the children. My mother in law had already missed visitations three times. The social worker is seeing how my mother in law is and you would think that she would be a little bit more firm as we go along because of

[my mother in laws] lack of cooperation, but she hasn't. So I feel that she isn't using her authority or being firm enough like she should. Maybe she only uses it when she wants.

This mother expected the worker to advocate and support her. The worker did set up a meeting with the caretaker; however, she did not advocate for the mother as the mother had hoped and expected.

Parents often reported that their worker was not entirely candid in the way they presented their role and purpose for being involved with the parent. Most parents stated that the social workers indicate that they are there to help; however, as stated by one parent, "*Yo me siento mas vigilada que ayudada*" ["I feel more watched over than helped"]. For many of the parents in this study it was their first interaction with the public child welfare system and they rely on what the worker said and trust their words. In an attempt to build rapport with families the workers may describe their role in a positive light; however, by not disclosing the major functions of their role with the family (protecting children as guided by current child welfare policy), child welfare workers do not properly inform parents of what they should expect from the worker and services.

> *La primera trabajadora me dijo que todo estaba bien. Que mi caso no era riesgoso porque mi hija con la que tuve el problema es una adolescente ya tiene 15 años y en este caso pues los niños ya hablan y que veía todo bien, pero que si me gustaría participar en un programa—ella nomás me dijo un programa ... Si me dijo que era voluntario, pero nunca le explican a uno que programa es, no sabe uno a que programa va a ir, y nadie se los explica. Yo le dije que estaba bien ... Nomás me dijo que si gustaba participar y que iba a mandar otra trabajadora. Yo lo hice para que vieran que no tengo nada que esconderles, que todo esta bien ... Pero ahora lo toman como un caso.*

> The first worker told me that everything was ok. That my case was not an at risk case because the daughter that I had a problem with was 15 years old and in this case all the kids [are older] and can speak and she said that everything was good. But she asked me if I would like to participate in a program—she only said a program ... She said that it was voluntary, but she never explained what program it was, we didn't know what program we were going to, and no one explains it. I said that it was ok ... She just said that if I would like to participate and that she was going to send another worker. I said yes so that they could see that I have nothing to hide, that everything is ok ... but now it's seen as a case.

The parent in this example was unaware that by agreeing to be part of this "program" she would have an open case with the public child welfare system. She was not informed that her involvement in this program would translate into monthly visits by a worker and weekly visits by an in-home counselor. Consequently, as parents have these negative experiences with the worker it is likely to impact their future interactions with systems of care. Families may elect to not seek help in a time of need or crisis in the future (Kerkorian, McKay, & Bannon, 2006).

Messages from Service Providers about Exercising Voice

Parents' interactions with other service providers validated their feelings about the power that workers hold in their cases. Parents often interact with several service providers when they have an open case with the public child welfare system (i.e., in addition to the worker, an in-home counselor through the Family Preservation program, therapist/counselor, and group facilitators). When parents shared their concerns with service providers they received mixed messages about what they should do if they are unsatisfied with the services they are receiving and about how they should interact with their worker. For example, one parent described how her in-home counselor (Family Preservation services) recommended that she contact the worker's supervisor, but she told her, "Don't focus on the worker, focus on the issue." The mother said that she felt that the in-home counselor had advised her to focus on the issue rather than the worker because if the worker saw it as a complaint then the worker would work against her. The mother said, "Yo lo tome como una advertencia que si me quejaba de la trabajadora me iba a perjudicar" ["I took as a warning that if I complained about the worker it was going to harm me"]. Another parent shared the feedback that was provided by a group facilitator.

> [The group facilitator] ... said you need to be cordial with your social worker because they hold some authority in returning your kids ... in the end it's up to the judge, but if the [worker] presents a good case against you then it's going to affect the decision that the judge makes.

Not only are parents aware of the power that their worker holds but it is confirmed by the comments or advise that the other services providers share. Thus, adding to the fear that parents experience and inhibiting them from speaking out if they are unsatisfied with aspects of their case. Moreover, parents learn from their interactions with their worker or with other service providers that they need to be cautious about what they say, how they say it, and to whom they say it. A climate of fear, intimidation, and silencing is fostered and sustained.

Exercising Voice: When is Voice Exercised? How Do Parents' Perceive Their Voice is Received by Workers?

As seen in the previous section, there are several factors that may inhibit parents from exercising their voice. However, parents do exercise their voice though they may be cautious about how and when it is done. Parents described many situations where they felt supported and understood by their worker, primarily when discussing their feelings about the problems the family was experiencing (e.g., substance abuse, domestic disputes).

WORKERS ASK FOR PARENTS' OPINIONS

On example of exercising voice occurs when workers ask for parents' opinions:

> When I relapsed, all those thoughts that were in my mind, I told her what I was feeling and ... how guilty I was and how ashamed I was and you know I believe that's why she gave me a second chance [with my kids].

This mother stated that her worker often inquired about her opinions and feelings about the case. She felt that her feelings were validated and she was heard by her worker. In a different case, the mother described that her worker had been very patient in listening to her concerns about her housing issues and how the worker took action and spoke to the landlord. The mother was very grateful for the worker's efforts to help her with her housing problem.

In contrast, some parents stated that workers rarely inquired about their opinions or feelings about the case: "No [my worker never asked about my opinions]. Yeah, I took the meeting or whatever kind of contact that we had as an opportunity to share my voice but I've never felt like she actually came to me to see how I'm doing or if I have any concerns or any needs or what ever." When parents expressed dissatisfaction with services, unmet service needs, or inquired about their case status, the worker's response was often characterized more negatively.

PARENTS INQUIRE ABOUT THEIR CASE

Some parents stated that they are ignored. "Cuando trato de hablar del tema se olvida la trabajadora del tema o se hace como que no me escucha o no me vuelve a contestar lo de mi pregunta" ["When I try to talk about the subject she forgets about it or she pretends not to hear me or she ignores my question again"]. Parents also revealed that in their attempts to obtain help the information that they disclose is used against them. In the next case, the parent shares what happened when she disclosed to her worker that she was HIV positive.

> ... last year I came out positive on HIV and I thought that the right thing was for me to ... tell my [worker] you know, I [wanted them] to test my girl because she was three months old. And instead of her reaction being it's ok you're not going to die or something ... she freaked out, she said oh my god you should leave your kids where they are. And from that

point on its been more like you have to educate yourself, are you under medication, are you doing this, don't touch the girls like that, your aunt gets mad when you kiss the kids too much, you can't feed your daughter from the same spoon. And things like that ... I feel like she attacks me more.

The mother disclosed her situation with the worker because she thought it was in the best interest of her child. However, revealing that she was HIV positive worked against her.

PARENTS DISCIPLINED INTO SILENCE

When parents' voices are ignored or used against them they tended to be silenced, that is, they tended not to voice their needs again as their efforts go without leading to a change. As a result some families went without getting their service needs met.

> I really got real depressed. I lost weight ... when they took my daughter away from me ... I was real depressed, but I didn't want to admit it ... but when you are by your self in the room and you just start crying and crying that's different ... I think the depression goes away, but it's always there. Just waiting for something ... I was never on medication ... I was scared to get treatment because ... I used to think that the [workers] were going to find out that I was on medication and that was going to make my case worse. I ... kept everything to my self. I couldn't tell the social worker ... I couldn't even tell my individual counselor because I didn't want them to report that. She did report that once, and, after that, I said "I'm never going to say nothing again" ... I saw the report in court and that was one more problem ... you know what I mean, you don't want any more problems ... if you have to fake it then that's what you have to do.

This mother went without appropriate mental health treatment because she knew that disclosing that information would keep her case open or hurt her case. Brown (2006) describes that many parents engage in emotional management to conceal their anger. In this case, the mother was concealing or "faking" that she was well and not experiencing any depression symptoms.

SELF-ADVOCACY AND PARENTAL ACTION

As seen in the case of Mrs. Gomez (noted in the opening quote of this article), parents do resist and take action. In the case of Mrs. Gomez, she and her husband had repeatedly stated that they had not physically abused their child. When their daughter was going to be adopted they decided to intervene and they kidnapped their daughter from the foster care parents. Although it was ultimately discovered that their daughter had a "brittle bone disease," as stated by Mrs. Gomez, ". . . everything that we had already been through was already there." Mrs. Gomez will never forget her experience with the public child welfare system and her struggle to be heard. Similarly, other parents attempt to resist being silenced by speaking to a supervisor. However, in most of the cases where parents shared that they sought out help from a supervisor the outcome did not lead to a positive change or action. One mother shared that on multiple occasions she attempted to call a supervisor, but she was simply unable to get through ["Hable al departamento para hablar con la supervisora pero nunca me la quisieron pasar"].

The next example was shared by the mother who is HIV positive. She shared her interactions with the supervisor and the outcome is that she is silenced.

> I had a [worker], the one that was racist and I felt discriminated because of my illness and I told her supervisor and then he was yelling. And I told him "Don't yell at me," and he said, "If you don't like it then we can end this conversation," and I said, "I just want to make my point across, I want you to hear me out." And he was yelling and he just hanged up on me. So then I thought I guess I'm going to have to talk to his supervisor. But I felt . . . like the [worker] didn't hear me, the supervisor didn't, what makes you think the other supervisor is going to hear me out . . . so I didn't do it.

One of the couples shared that they had seen a supervisor to address a concern and the supervisor had recommended to them that they write a detailed letter and submit it to the department. The parents exercised their voice by speaking to a supervisor and although the supervisor recommended that they make the complaint more formal. Both parents had limited English skills and they did not feel competent to write the type of letter that the supervisor had suggested.

In the next case the mother found that she was heard and she was able to regain her children and get a new worker assigned to her. The difference was that she had a network that was there to support her and advocate for her.

> *Yo hable con la supervisora, fue mi trabajadora la del [programa de violencia domestica] ese día. Ella siempre a ido con migo . . . [Ella va con migo] para sentirme mas segura. Porque como la supervisora no hablaba español, si pusieron una traductora [pero] las cosas que no se decían bien la [trabajador del programa de violencia domestica me las] explicaba bien. Porque muchas veces cuando nomás hablan ingles y no español confunden las palabras. Lo que pasa fue que casi ya iban a ser 3 meses de cuando me iban a regresar los niños. Y a mí eso fue lo que me dijeron cuando yo firme . . . Yo le dije que me habían recomendado*

que hablara con la supervisora del caso porque yo también ya tenía casi un mes que no miraba a los niños porque no los traía el papa. Todo eso, hable de todo lo que no me gustaba. Y si me hicieron caso, a la semana me cambiaron la trabajadora.

I talked to the supervisor, my worker from the domestic violence program went with me that day. She always goes with me. [She goes with me] so that I feel more confident. Because since the supervisor does not speak English, they did have a translator but the things that are not translated well the worker from the DV program would explain them to me. Because many times when they only speak English and not Spanish they confuse the words. What happened was that it was going to be three months since they were going to return my kids. That's what they told me when I signed the paperwork ... I told them that it had been suggested to me that I speak to the case supervisor because I also had about one month that I hadn't seen my kids because the dad wouldn't bring them. I talked about everything that I didn't like. And they listened to me. In a week they had changed my worker.

Having support from someone who is well informed about how systems work helped this mother to be heard and the interaction with the supervisor resulted in an actual change. Similarly, Marcenko and Striepe (1997) found that substance abuse treatment facilities provide women with much needed support network. In addition, this mother speaks to the barrier that language plays in being heard and about the incompetence of people who translate for such families. Unfortunately, not many parents had the type of support that this mother had.

In the following example, the interview was completed with both parents. The father speaks to the need for guidance and support from someone who knows the system.

Pues [yo le recomendaría] a los otros padres que ... si sus trabajadores no les están ayudando que los cambien. Pero desde el principio no cuando ya se va acabar el caso como el de nosotros. Nosotros no sabíamos ... nunca nos orientaron con nada de esto. Si a nosotros nos hubieran dicho que si tu trabajador no te esta ayudando cámbialo o [nos] hubiera explicado [el proceso] poquito, créame que desde el principio hubiéramos hecho algo. Si porque uno va con los ojos cerrados, vendados ... uno va a las cortes va haciendo lo que los trabajadores te dicen que hagas. Te dicen da un paso y ya uno lo tiene que dar con los ojos cerrados. Y que dale para la derecha, dale para la izquierda, y uno lo tiene que hacer. Pero si alguien nos orienta desde antes ... desde que empieza el caso, no mira va a pasar así ... Ósea, si tu miras como que el [trabajador] no te esta ayudando que el esta haciendo mal tu habla y dile. Y si sientes que de veras no te ayuda ... apela para que lo cambien ... ¿Me entiendes? ¿Pero si uno no dice nada pues donde va a quedar uno?

No te van ayudar. Va a pasar lo que [los trabajadores] quieren que pase ... ¿Porque? porque uno [no sabe que hacer].

Well [I would recommend] to other parents that ... if their workers are not helping them they should change them. But from the beginning, not when the case is going to end like ours. We didn't know ... no one ever oriented us about the any of this. If someone would have told us that, if our worker wasn't helping us, we should change him or if someone would have explained [the process] a little bit, believe me that from the beginning we would have done something. Because it's like we are doing everything with your eyes closed, blind folded ... we go to the courts and we do what the workers tell us do to. They tell you take a step and you have to do it with your eyes closed. And go to the right, go to the left, and you just have to do it. But if someone had oriented us before ... when the case started, no, look, it's going to be like this ... If you see that your [worker] is not helping you, that he is doing his job wrong, you speak out and tell him. And if you feel that he is not helping you ... make an appeal, so that they will change him ... Do you understand? But if you don't say anything, what's going to happen? They are not going to help you. What [the workers] want will happen ... Why? Because we [don't know what to do].

These parents have been supportive to one another throughout the process. However, as described by the father, they did not know what to expect and he felt like he was blind folded through most of the process. He believes that if there had been someone to "orient" them their experience would have been different.

Many of the parents in this study often felt powerless and voiceless. However, the well-being of their family is important to them; therefore, parents frequently inquired about the status of their case or advocated for their family if they were unsatisfied with the services or worker. The reception that parents experienced when they exercised their voice played a significant role in whether they continued to exercise their voice. When parents were continuously ignored or when they realized that the information they disclosed was used against them, parents often discontinued voicing their needs, expectations, and dissatisfaction with services. At times parents' concerns were validated; however, in such instances it rarely resulted in change. Some parents who were unsatisfied with the worker's response would attempt to contact a supervisor, but too often their efforts did not lead to change except in the case where the parent brought in a support agent. This finding is significant because it is not enough to have a spouse or family member who is there advocating with the parent. Having someone who knows the system is crucial to facilitating positive change. In other words, it is not enough to have a dancing partner. The parent needs to have a dance instructor, or someone that knows the system, by the parent's side, teaching them the steps to advocate within the public child welfare system.

LIMITATIONS

This study has limitations related to the sampling. The study is based on a convenient sample and parents were only recruited in one child welfare office in Southern California; therefore, generalizability is limited. Only parents' experiences are included in this article. Because cases were ongoing parent–worker dyads were not interviewed, in order to protect parents. Interviewing parent–worker dyads in ongoing cases may prevent parents and workers from freely sharing information. Future studies should include multiple perspectives. It is important to note that this study examines, from the parent's perspectives, the experiences of Mexican families with a history of immigration, a population that has not been well studied within child welfare research.

IMPLICATIONS FOR SOCIAL WORK PRACTICE AND POLICY

Policy changes and practice models that promote the provision of family-centered and culturally and linguistically relevant services are needed and should be supported within the public child welfare system. This study finds that parents' frequently voiced their needs during monthly social worker visits. However, Mexican parents' interactions and experiences with their worker coupled with their fear of losing their children and immigration consequences tended to silence them thus preventing effective parent engagement. To address this issue and to promote effective service delivery and outcomes, day-to-day parent-worker interactions need to be grounded in the principles of family centered practices.

It is imperative that social workers are trained to provide culturally responsive services and utilize empowerment models effectively to facilitate the *active participation* of parents in the case process. When families are involved with the public child welfare system the aim is to create a change that will promote children's (and families') well-being. If families are actively engaged in this process they may be able to acquire skills and knowledge that they can use in the future when they encounter additional needs. Parents' interactions with child welfare workers can significantly influence their future help seeking behavior (Diorio, 1992) and how they perceive their ability to change their circumstances.

Given the lack of success that the child welfare system has demonstrated in reducing the overrepresentation of ethnic minority families in foster care and persistent disparities in care (Hill, 2003; Wulczyn & Lery, 2007), it is crucial that the provision of culturally responsive services tailored to culturally diverse families be core to child welfare workers' training rather than a peripheral issue. Grounding practices in families' cultural practices along with understanding other contextual factors such as their immigration history is fundamental to engaging families in responsive ways. For example, workers' interactions with Mexican/Latino families need to be responsive to the value of *personalismo. Personalismo* involves more intimate interactions between the service provider as a means to building trust and rapport (Committee for Hispanic Children and Families, 2004); that is, workers may need to disclose personal information (more than they regularly would) or share stories with the parent in order to establish a good relationship. In this study the lack of cultural relevance in services is illustrated in parents' description of the lack of clarity about their worker's role and unmet expectations. The parent–worker relationship has to be a trustworthy partnership where the worker and parent know each other well—from this space both parties can work toward addressing the needs of the family. Similarly, linguistically appropriate services are also needed. Study participants shared the lack of proficient translators.

As Latino immigrant families may not be familiar with systems of care in the United States informal and formal sources of support are needed to guide parents and inform parents of their rights. Interventions that provide informal support and advocacy to parents (such as parent-to-parent role modeling, foster parent-to-parent dyad relationships, and mutual-aid/support peer groups) should continue to be supported. Such programs can help parents feel more informed and connected to their case process. In addition, to providing informal support and information, families should also have access to formal advocates as this study finds that having support from someone who knows the system is important to being heard and addressing families' needs.

Structural factors such as large case loads, extreme needs of families served, and paperwork can restrict workers' engagement with families. Study findings suggest that the integration of parents' voice (their opinions and point of view) is necessary to effectively meet the needs of families served by this institution. Therefore, it is crucial that the public child welfare agencies adopt a mission and implement policies that will systematically promote and facilitate workers authentic and collaborative interactions with families. Parents' feedback should be encouraged and solicited to inform the development of child welfare interventions and to evaluate existing interventions. Families and workers must effectively engage in the creation of an environment compatible with human needs in order to promote social justice (Gutiérrez et al., 2003) and minimize the disparities Latino children and families experience while maximizing the effectiveness of the service plan.

REFERENCES

Alpert, L. T., & Brinter, P. A. (2009). Measuring parent engagement in foster care. *Social Work Research, 33*(3), 135–145.

Alzate, M. M., & Rosenthal, J. A. (2009). Gender and ethnic differences for Hispanic children referred to child protective services. *Children and Youth Services Review, 31*, 1–7.

American Humane Association (2008). *Family group decision making in child welfare: Purpose, values and processes.* Retrieved from http://www.americanhumane.org/assets/docs/protecting–children/PC–fgdm–statements.pdf

Baca Zinn, M. (1994). Adaptation and continuity in Mexican-origin families. In R. L. Taylor (ed.), *Minority families in the United States: A multicultural perspective* (pp. 66–82). Upper Saddle River, New Jersey: Prentice Hall.

Brown, D. J. (2006). Working the system: Re–thinking the institutionally organized role of mothers and the reduction of "risk" in child protection work. *Social Problems, 53*, 352–370.

Cauce, A. M., & Domenech-Rodriguez, M. (2000). Latino families: Myths and realities. In J. M. Contreras, K. A. Kerns, & A. M. Neal-Barnett (eds.), *Latino children and families in the United States* (pp. 3–25). Westport, CT: Praeger Publishers.

Charmaz, K. (2005). Grounded theory in the 21st Century: Applications for advancing social justice studies. In N. K. Denzin & Y. S. Lincoln (eds.), *The Sage handbook of qualitative research* (pp. 507–535). Thousand Oaks, CA: Sage Publications.

Charmaz, K. (2006). *Constructing grounded theory: A practical guide through qualitative analysis.* Thousand Oaks, CA: Sage Publications.

Church, W. T. (2006). From start to finish: The duration of Hispanic children in out–of–home placements. *Children and Youth Services Review, 28*, 1007–1023.

Church, W. T., Gross, E., & Baldwin, J. (2005). Maybe ignorance is not always bliss: The disparate treatment of Hispanics within the child welfare system. *Children and Youth Services Review, 27*, 1279–1292.

Cohen, E., & Canan, L. (2006). Closer to home: Parent mentors in child welfare. *Child Welfare, 85*, 867–884.

Committee for Hispanic Children and Families (2004). *Creating a Latino child welfare agenda: A strategic framework for change.* New York, NY: Committee for Hispanic Children and Families, Inc.

Corby, B., Millar, M., & Young, L. (1996). Parental participation in child protection work: Rethinking the rhetoric. *British Journal of Social Work, 26*, 475–492.

Crampton, D. (2006). When do social workers and family members try family group decision making? A process evaluation. *International Journal of Child and Family Welfare, 3*, 131–144.

Dawson, K., & Berry, M. (2002). Engaging families in child welfare services: An evidence–based approach to best practice. *Child Welfare, 8*, 293–317.

deBoer, C., & Coady, N. (2007). Good helping relationships in child welfare: Learning from stories of success. *Child and Family Social Work, 12*, 32–42.

Diorio, W. D. (1992). Parental perceptions of the authority of public child welfare caseworkers. *Families in Society, 73*, 222–235.

Dumbrill, G. C. (2006). Parental experiences of child protection intervention: A qualitative study. *Child Abuse and Neglect, 30*, 27–37.

Fontes, L. A. (2002). Child disciplinary and physical abuse in immigrant Latino families: Reducing violence and misunderstandings. *Journal of Counseling and Development, 80*, 37–47.

Frame, L., Conley, A., & Berrick, J. D. (2006). "The real work is what they do together": Peer support and birth parent change. *Families in Society, 87*, 509–520.

Garland, A. F., Landsverk, J. A., & Lau, A. S. (2003). Racial/ethnic disparities in mental health service use among children in foster care. *Children and Youth Services Review, 25*, 491–507.

Gutiérrez, L. M., Parsons, R. J., & Cox, E. O. (2003). *Empowerment in social work practice: A source book.* Stamford, CT: Wadsworth/Thomas Learning Center.

Hill, R. B. (2003). *Synthesis of research on disproportionality in child welfare: An update.* Washington, DC: Casey–CSSP Alliance for Racial Equity in Child Welfare.

Hines, A. M., Lemon, K., Wyatt, P., & Merdinger, J. (2004). Factors related to the disproportionate involvement of children of color in the child welfare system: A review and emerging themes. *Children and Youth Service Review, 26*, 507–527.

Hirschman, A. O. (1970). *Exit, voice, and loyalty.* Cambridge, MA: Harvard University Press.

Holland, S. (2000). The assessment relationship: Interactions between social workers and parents in child protection assessments. *British Journal of Social Work, 30*, 149–163.

Kapp, S., & Propp, J. (2002). Client satisfaction methods: Input from parents with children in foster care. *Child and Adolescent Social Work, 19*, 227–245.

Kapp, S., & Vela, R. (2004). The unheard client: Assessing the satisfaction of parents of children in foster care. *Child and Family Social Work, 9*, 197–206.

Kemp, S. P., Marcenko, M. O., Hoagwood, K., & Vesneski, W. (2009). Engaging parents in child welfare services: Bridging family needs and child welfare mandates. *Child Welfare, 88*, 101–126.

Kerkorian, D., McKay, M., & Bannon, W. (2006). Seeking help a second time: Parents'/caregivers' characterizations of previous experiences with mental health services for their children and perceptions of barriers to future use. *American Journal of Orthopsychiatry, 76*, 161–166.

Lee, C. D., & Ayón, C. (2004). Is the client–worker relationship associates with better outcomes in mandated child abuse cases? *Research on Social Work Practice, 14*, 351–357.

Lee, C. D., & Ayón, C. (2007). Family preservation: The parents' perceptions. *Family Preservation Journal, 10*, 42–61.

Linares, O., Montalto, D., Li, M., & Oza, V. S. (2006). A promising parenting intervention in foster care. *Journal of Consulting and Clinical Psychology, 74*, 32–41.

Loue, S., Faust, M., & Bunce, A. (2000). The effects of immigration and welfare reform legislation on immigrants' access to health care, Cuyahoga, and Lorain Counties. *Journal of Immigrant Health, 2*, 23–30.

Marcenko, M. O., & Striepe, M. I. (1997). A look at family reunification through the eyes of mothers. *Community Alternatives, 9*, 33–48.

Petr, C. G., & Entriken, C. (1995). Service system barriers to reunification. *Families in Society, 76*, 523–533.

Snowden, L. R., & Yamada, A. M. (2005). Cultural differences in access to care. *Annual Review of Clinical Psychology, 1*, 143–166.

Strauss, A., & Corbin, J. (1990). *Basics of qualitative research: Grounded theory procedures and techniques.* London, England: Sage Publications.

Suleiman Gonzalez, L. P. (2004). Five commentaries: Looking toward the future. *Future of Children, 14*(1), 184–189.

United States Department of Health and Human Services (US DHHS). Administration on Children, Youth and Families (1997). *Child Maltreatment 1995*. Washington, DC: US Government Printing Office.

United States Department of Health and Human Services (US DHHS). Administration of Children, Youth and Families (2007). *Child Maltreatment 2005*. Washington, DC: US Government Printing Office.

Wulczyn, F. W., & Lery, B. (2007). *Racial disparity in foster care admissions*. Chicago, IL: Chapin Hall Center for Children at the University of Chicago.

Yatchmenoff, D. K. (2005). Measuring client engagement from the client's perspective in nonvoluntary child protective services. *Research on Social Work Practice, 15*(2), 84–96.

A Review of Family-Based Mental Health Treatments That May Be Suitable for Children in Immigrant Families Involved in the Child Welfare System

KYA FAWLEY-KING

Children from immigrant families who are involved in the child welfare system face unique circumstances that can be harmful to their mental health. To date, there are no documented mental health treatment programs designed specifically for this population. However, there are family-based mental health treatments for immigrant families. Additionally, several evidence-based mental health treatments have been successfully applied to children in the child welfare system. A review of both types of treatments shows that these interventions have many positive aspects that may fit the needs of both maltreating and immigrant families. It is possible that these interventions could be successfully modified to aid children from immigrant families involved in the child welfare system.

Children who are victims of maltreatment often suffer from mental health problems. Estimates of the prevalence of emotional and behavioral disorders among children in the child welfare system (CWS) range from 40% to 80% (Burns, Phillips, Wagner, Barth, Kolko, et al., 2004; Clausen, Landsverk, Ganger, Chadwick, & Litronik, 1998; Garland, Landsverk, Hough, & Ellis-MacLeod, 1996). While there are currently no estimates of the prevalence of mental health problems among children of immigrants in the CWS, these children face many obstacles that can be detrimental to their mental health.

Children in the CWS have frequently been exposed to poverty, domestic violence, parental mental illness and parental substance abuse, and any child exposed to these risk factors has an increased likelihood of developing mental health problems (Kerker & Dore, 2006). Children from immigrant families are often exposed to these risk factors as well. For example, in 2006, 51% of children of immigrants lived in families with incomes below the federal poverty level (Fortuny, Capps, Simms, & Chaudry, 2009). Additionally, some researchers have found high rates of intimate partner violence in Hispanic, South Asian, and Korean immigrant families (Raj & Sliverman, 2002). Furthermore, for some immigrant families, the experience of migrating to another country can be traumatic enough to cause the parents to develop symptoms of post-traumatic stress disorder (PTSD) (Dettlaff, Earner, & Phillips, 2009; Segal & Mayadas, 2005).

However, immigrant families that are involved in the CWS also face unique stressors that can be harmful to the children's mental health. Chronic poverty is especially detrimental for children (Bolger, Patterson, Thompson, & Kupersmidt, 1995), but undocumented immigrant parents may have a harder time alleviating their poverty because they are not eligible for government assistance programs such as Temporary Aid for Needy Families (TANF) and Supplemental Nutrition Assistance Program (SNAP).

Also, acculturation can be a stressful process for many immigrant families, especially if the children acculturate at a faster rate than the parents. Due to the fact that children of immigrants must attend U.S. schools, they frequently learn English and American customs more quickly than their parents (Portes & Rumbaut, 2001; Sluzki, 1979). Conflict can arise if the children start to follow American customs that are in opposition with their parents' traditional views about how children should behave (Portes & Rumbaut, 2001; Sluzki, 1979). There is some evidence that family conflicts resulting from acculturation gaps can lead to depression in youth (Ying & Han, 2007).

Most immigrant families living in the United States are non-White (Fortuny et al., 2009). Both non-White immigrant youth and native-born youth from racial/ethnic minority backgrounds may encounter discrimination. However, for non-White immigrant youth who were part of the racial majority in their country of origin, the transition to minority status and subsequent encounters with racism may come as a shock. Furthermore, immigrant youth may face xenophobia and discriminatory attitudes towards immigrants in general.

In addition to possibly being victims of discrimination, youth in immigrant families who enter the CWS have been maltreated. Immigrant communities frequently have a culture of silence (Segal & Mayadas, 2005) and mistrust authorities (Chahine & Van Straaten, 2005). It is possible that cases of child abuse and neglect in these communities are not brought to the attention of authorities unless the cases are severe (Dettlaff, Earner, & Phillips, 2009). For example, Hispanic youth from immigrant families are more likely to enter the CWS due to sexual abuse (Dettlaff et al., 2009) and to be removed from home due to sexual abuse (Vericker, Kuehn, & Capps, 2007) than Hispanic children who were born in the United States.

While being removed from home and placed into foster care can be traumatic for any youth (Kerker & Dore, 2006), it may be especially traumatic for children of immigrants. First of all, the removal may be the *second* time that these children are separated from their homes and family members. Children who are immigrants themselves will have already left their country of origin, and in the case of refugees, they may have been forced to leave against their will (Segal & Mayadas, 2005). Additionally, families sometimes immigrate in stages—one or both parents may immigrate first, and wait until they are financially secure before bringing all of the children to the United States (Garcia 2001 as cited in Dettlaff et al., 2009). Thus, children of immigrants who are placed in foster care may have been separated from their mothers or fathers one or more times before.

Secondly, immigrants may have no extended family in the United States (Segal & Mayadas, 2005), in which case it may be impossible to place a child from an immigrant family into kinship care. One study of 20,406 children in Texas' foster care system found that Hispanic children from immigrant families were significantly less likely to be placed in kinship care than Hispanic children whose parents were born in the United States (Vericker, Kuehn, & Capps, 2007).

Furthermore, some immigrant families live in neighborhoods with large numbers of other immigrant families from the same country of origin, and if a child is placed in foster care outside of this type of neighborhood, the child will lose the social support that the child's former community offered. Thus, when children from immigrant families are placed in out-of-home care, they may be forced to adjust to living with an unfamiliar family in an unfamiliar neighborhood where the culture is different from their own.

Finally, approximately one third of children of immigrants have parents who are not citizens (Fortuny et al., 2009), and some of these parents may be undocumented. Placement into foster care may be especially traumatic for children whose parents are undocumented, because they may fear that their parents will be deported before reunification can occur.

PURPOSE

Although children from immigrant families in the CWS face unique circumstances that can be harmful to their mental health, there have not been any documented mental health treatments designed specifically for this population. However, it is possible that existing mental health treatments could be adapted to meet the needs of these families. First, this article will review family-based mental health treatments for immigrants and evaluate their compatibility for families involved in CWS. Next, this article will review evidence-based mental health treatments that are effective for maltreated children and their caregivers, and research on the application of these interventions with families in other countries as well as ethnic minority families living in the United States. This article will then discuss reasons the treatments may or may not be effective for immigrant families. The last treatment reviewed in this article will be an intervention that has been tested with both maltreating and immigrant families. Finally, this article will conclude with an analysis of how the reviewed treatments could be adapted for different types of immigrant families with CWS involvement and suggestions for future research.

The reviews in this article are not exhaustive. Rather they showcase interventions that either: a) have a well-developed parent component, b) have strong research support, or c) are specifically designed for groups that have not traditionally been the focus of mental health treatment programs (such as Asians or children living in foster care). More information on treatment programs for immigrant families is available from the National Child Traumatic Stress Network (2005) and is reported in Rousseau, Benoit, Gauthier, Lacroix, Alain, et al. (2007). Additional information on evidence-based mental health treatment for children in the CWS is reported in Shipman and Taussig (2009).

FAMILY-BASED MENTAL HEALTH TREATMENTS FOR IMMIGRANT FAMILIES

Entre Dos Mundos (Between Two Worlds)

The goal of Entre Dos Mundos is to help Hispanic immigrant families handle acculturative stress and prevent externalizing-behavior problems in adolescents ages 12 to 18 years. The program consists of eight lessons that are delivered weekly to a group of 810 families. At least one parent and one adolescent are expected to come to each meeting. The lessons all focus on aspects of acculturative stress such as balancing demands of two cultures, cultural conflict within the family, and discrimination (Smokowski & Bacallao, 2009).

Smokowski and Bacallao (2009) examined the effectiveness of this program when it was delivered to 88 primarily Mexican immigrant families living in North Carolina. The researchers found that, in families who attended more than four sessions, the adolescents had significant decreases in aggression, and symptoms of oppositional defiant and attention deficit disorders. Additionally, the families had significant improvements in adaptability and biculturalism.

Familias Unidas (Families United)

Similar to Entre Dos Mundos, Familias Unidas is designed to prevent externalizing-behavior problems in adolescents from immigrant families. However, rather than focusing on acculturative stress, this intervention focuses on increasing parental involvement in children's lives. Familias Unidas has been designed for youth in middle school and it also seeks to reduce drug use and risky sexual behaviors (Tapia, Schwartz, Lopez, & Pantin, 2006).

Familias Unidas is a 9-month intervention with several different stages. In the first stage, the facilitators work very hard to engage the families by calling them and conducting a home visit. During these interactions with the family, the facilitators address concerns about the intervention and explain how it can specifically help the family. When parents begin the treatment, they are taught that their adolescents live in three worlds: family, peers, and school, and that it is important for parents to be involved in each of the worlds. Next, the treatment focuses on the "family world" and parents are taught how to communicate in a non-judgmental style and how to use behavior management techniques to discipline their children. In the stage that addresses the "school world" a counselor from a middle school comes and teaches the parents about the United States school system. In the "peer world" stage, parents plan an outing with their adolescent and one of their adolescent's friends and his or her parent/s. Finally, parents learn how to talk about substance abuse and sexual behavior with their adolescents in a supportive manner (Tapia, Schwartz, Lopez, & Pantin, 2006).

Preliminary research on this intervention has found that it has positive outcomes. In one randomized controlled trial with 167 Hispanic immigrant families from several different countries, families in the intervention group showed significant improvement in parental involvement and decreases in adolescent externalizing problems compared to families in the control group who did not receive any intervention. Additionally, parents who were the least involved with their adolescents prior to the intervention attended the most sessions and gained the most from treatment (Pantin, Coatsworth, Feaster, Newman, Briones, et al., 2003). In a second study with 266 Hispanic families randomly assigned to either Familias Unidas with PATH (an intervention designed to help parents and adolescents speak about HIV) or English for Speakers of Other Languages with PATH, or English for Speakers of Other Languages with HeartPower! (an intervention designed to promote physical health), the adolescent participants in Familias Unidas had the biggest decreases in drug use and risky sexual behavior (Pantin et al., 2005 as cited in Tapia et al., 2006).

Mental Health for Immigrants Program (MHIP)

Unlike Entre Dos Mundos and Familias Unidas, MHIP is delivered to children in schools with four optional sessions for parents. The goal of MHIP is to decrease symptoms of depression and PTSD among immigrant children in grades 3 through 8 who have been exposed to violence. Children attend eight group therapy sessions that follow the Cognitive Behavioral Intervention for Trauma in Schools (CBITS) model. The CBITS program teaches children methods from cognitive behavioral therapy that help individuals cope with upsetting memories and feelings of grief.

The group sessions for parents cover a variety of topics. Parents discuss the difficulties of the immigration process and are taught about how trauma can affect children. These sessions also provide psycho-education about the CBITS model and information on parenting practices. MHIP includes an in-service training session for teachers, which provides instructions about how children may react to trauma, and how to recognize possible symptoms of PTSD and depression (Kataoka, Stein, Jaycox, Wong, Escudero, et al., 2003).

MHIP was first implemented in the Los Angeles Unified School District and offered to Spanish, Armenian, Korean, and Russian immigrant children (Stein et al., 2003). However, the published research only reports results for the Hispanic immigrant participants in the intervention. The pilot study included 198 Hispanic immigrant students from 9 different elementary and middle schools. Forty-six of these students were assigned to the waitlist control condition. After adjusting for participants' initial symptom levels, students in the experimental group had significantly fewer symptoms of depression than students in the control group 3 months after the intervention ended. Furthermore, when the outcomes of the students who began the study with symptoms in the clinical range were compared, students who received the intervention had significantly greater decreases in both depression and PTSD (Kataoka et al., 2003).

Strengthening of Intergenerational/Intercultural Ties in Immigrant Chinese American Families (SITICAF)

SITICAF is an 8-week parent-training program for Chinese parents who have migrated to the United States. The 2-hour classes cover many topics: cross-cultural encounters, ethnic identity formation, cultural differences, child development, parenting practices such as active listening and limit setting, and handling stress. The classes are delivered in Mandarin, and the class format includes lectures, group exercises and homework (Ying, 1999).

This intervention has not been researched extensively, but a pilot study with 15 parents found that participation in SITICAF lead to increased sense of parenting responsibility, control of the child, and improvements in the parent-child relationship. While the intervention did not significantly affect children's mental health, the quality of the parent-child relationship at the end of the program and at 3-months follow-up was significantly related to the child's self esteem (Ying, 1999).

COMPATIBILITY OF FAMILY-BASED MENTAL HEALTH INTERVENTIONS FOR IMMIGRANTS WITH FAMILIES IN THE CHILD WELFARE SYSTEM

While none of the aforementioned programs have been tested with children from immigrant families in the CWS, there are many aspects of these interventions that indicate they may be effective for this unique population. For example, the main benefits of all of these programs are that they address acculturation stress, are delivered in the families' native languages, and tackle intergenerational cultural conflicts. Mental health treatments provided to children and families in the CWS typically do not address these issues. If maltreatment in an immigrant family stems from difficulty coping with the children's more rapid acculturation or with other aspects of the transition to life in the United States, then these programs may be superior to therapies that focus on other causes of maltreated children's emotional and behavioral problems.

Another benefit of these programs is that they are all group-based. Participating in therapy groups gives both parents and children the chance to meet other people from immigrant families who are coping with similar problems. The opportunity to meet other people and possibly make new friends may also be especially beneficial to maltreating parents. Parents who are neglectful typically have smaller social networks and fewer friends or relatives who live nearby than parents who are not neglectful. Meanwhile parents who are physically abusive have fewer close relationships than non-maltreating parents (Coohey, 1996).

The fact that all of the programs involve the children's biological parents is another sign that these programs may be helpful for families involved in the CWS. Most children who have contact with this system are not removed from home (Barth, Landsverk, Chamberlain, Reid, Rolls, et al., 2005) and most children who are placed in foster care are reunified with their biological parents within 2 years (American Academy of Child and Adolescent Psychiatry, 2005). Thus, it is very important to include parents in treatment when providing mental health services to children in child welfare.

Despite their potential effectiveness, these programs also have several potential limitations. For example, the children in the studies of these programs did not necessarily have mental health problems. Children in the CWS have high rates of psychological disorders (Burns et al., 2004; Clausen et al., 1998; Garland et al., 1996) and it is possible that these programs would not be able to effectively reduce their psychiatric distress.

Also, all of the families in the research studies volunteered to participate. Yet, families in the CWS may be mandated to attend treatment programs (Barth et al., 2005), and researchers have found that they are more likely than non-maltreating families to drop out of treatment prematurely (Lau & Weisz, 2003). The interventions designed for immigrant families could be less effective with families in which the parents were not participating out of their own free will. However, it is also possible that the intensive engagement strategies used in Familias Unidas could significantly improve the retention of these families in treatment.

As reflected in the reviews, research on most of these programs is limited in number and methodological rigor to one or two observational studies with the exception of Familias Unidas which has been evaluated in two randomized controlled trials (Tapia et al., 2006). Before applying these treatments to immigrant families in the CWS it would be useful to conduct additional trials of their effectiveness.

Finally, all of these interventions are created for children living with their biological parents, and both Entre Dos Mundos and Familias Unidas are designed to address conflicts that occur between immigrant parents and their children when the children acculturate more quickly to the United States (Smokowski & Bacallao, 2009; Tapia et al., 2006). Yet if children from immigrant families are not brought to the attention of the CWS unless the incidents of abuse and neglect are severe, as has been hypothesized (Dettlaff et al., 2009), then it is likely that a high proportion will end up in foster care. Furthermore, these children may be placed in families of a different ethnicity. Or, they may be placed with caregivers who are of the same ethnicity, but the caregivers may have lived in the United States for longer than the child and may be more accustomed to United States culture. Thus, these foster families may need interventions that teach the caregivers about the child's culture and heritage, or that help them cope with conflicts between highly acculturated parents and less-acculturated children.

EVIDENCE-BASED MENTAL HEALTH TREATMENTS FOR FAMILES IN THE CHILD WELFARE SYSTEM

Trauma-Focused Cognitive Behavioral Therapy (TF-CBT)

TF-CBT is a treatment for sexually abused children ages 3 to 18 years that contains a mixture of cognitive behavior therapy and techniques used to treat PTSD. It is conducted in 12 to 16 sessions with both the child and the non-offending parent. The child and the parent are typically seen separately except for three joint sessions. The intervention covers parenting skills, common reactions to childhood trauma, relaxation and desensitization techniques, identifying relationships between thoughts, feelings, and behaviors, using positive self-talk, and problem solving. The child is asked to write a story about the trauma experienced, and the therapist helps the child identify and challenge the child's cognitive distortions related to the experience. The child also reads the trauma narrative to the parent, and they work on improving their communication. They also generate ways to help keep the child safe in the future (Cohen, Mannarino, Murray, & Igelman, 2006).

At least six randomized controlled trials have examined the effectiveness of TF-CBT and have found that TF-CBT was superior to non-directive supportive therapies, and Rogerian style therapies, at reducing symptoms of PTSD and behavioral problems (Cohen, Mannarino, Murray, & Igelman, 2006). Additionally, TF-CBT is one of the primary treatments used in the Community Outreach Program-Esperanza offered by the National Crime Victims Research and Treatment Center at the Medical University of South Carolina (Charleston, SC). This program provides case management and mental health services to children who have been victims of crime. Many of the program recipients are immigrant families from Mexico (De Arellano, Waldrop, Deblinger, Cohen, & Mannarino, 2005; De Arellano, Ko, Danielson, & Sprague, 2008).

The experience of working with these families has lead to the development of a modified version of TF-CBT for Hispanics. Some of the modifications include providing a more thorough explanation of therapy in the psycho-education component, and reframing the discipline techniques as ways to increase respect because Hispanic parents may expect their children to be more respectful of adult authority than do White American parents (De Arellano, 2009). TF-CBT has also been modified for African refugees (Murray, Cohen, Ellis, & Mannarino, 2008) and for use in the Netherlands, Germany, Norway, Russia, Pakistan, Palestine/Israel, Sri Lanka, Indonesia and Thailand (De Arellano et al., 2008). The outcomes of these modified versions have not yet been published.

Parent–Child Interaction Therapy (PCIT)

In contrast to TF-CBT, which addresses internalizing problems, PCIT is a treatment for children age 2 to 6 years with behavioral disorders. PCIT has two phases: child-directed interaction (CDI) and parent-directed interaction (PDI), and it is implemented in 14 1-hour sessions. During each session the child is in a playroom with one of the parents (usually the mother), and the parent has an electronic ear "bug" through which the parent receives instructions from a therapist who is watching the activities in the playroom through a one-way mirror. The goal of the CDI phase is to teach the parent and child how to interact in a positive manner. The parent learns to let the child control the play session and to praise the child effectively. In the PDI phase, the parent learns how to give clear instructions to the child and how to apply appropriate consequences for misbehavior (Chaffin, Silovsky, Funderburk, Valle, Brestan, et al., 2004; Herschell, Calzada, Eyberg, & McNeil, 2002; Timmer, Urquiza, Zebell, & McGrath, 2005).

Research on PCIT has found that it improves maltreating parents' interactions with their children, reduces children's symptoms of externalizing disorders, and lowers the risk of re-abuse (Chaffin et al., 2004; Timmer et al., 2005). Besides being successful with maltreating families, it has also been found to be an effective treatment for foster families in which the caregivers are having difficulties coping with children with behavior problems (Timmer, Urquiza, Herschell, McGrath, Zebell, et al., 2006; Timmer, Urquiza, & Zebell, 2006).

PCIT has also been successfully adapted and applied to children living in other countries. For example, Leung and colleagues (2009) studied the effectiveness of PCIT with Chinese families living in Hong Kong. The assessment measurements were translated into Chinese and the therapists spoke Cantonese, but no other modifications were made to the program. The researchers found that the 48 families in the intervention group had significantly greater improvements in parenting practices, parenting stress, and child behavior than the 62 families in the comparison group who did not receive treatment.

When PCIT was implemented in Puerto Rico the treatment received more modifications. In addition to translating the assessment measures and providing the treatment in Spanish, treatment providers modified the program for Puerto Rican children by working to establish a warm personal relationship with the mothers, using idiomatic expressions, and helping mothers figure out how to involve the extended families in treatment. The modified version was only tested with nine Puerto Rican families, but it led to improvements in the children's behavior problems and the parents' use of discipline techniques (Matos, Torres, Santiago, Jurado, & Rodriguez, 2006).

PCIT has also been modified for Mexican American families. The adapted version—Guiando a Niños Activos (GANA [Guiding Active Children])—has a more extensive engagement protocol than typical PCIT. The protocol was changed because research suggests that even if Mexican American mothers are interested in the treatment, they may not participate if the child's father and grandparents are opposed to it. The more extensive engagement protocol includes contact with the fathers and extended family members in order to discuss any reservations they have about the treatment. Because having a child with mental health problems can be seen as shameful in the Mexican American community, the GANA program is advertised as an "educational" treatment and the therapists are called *maestros* (*teachers*). Additionally, the handouts for the GANA program have been translated into Spanish and re-written in simpler language for parents with lower education levels (McCabe, Yeh, Garland, Lau, & Chavez, 2005).

A pilot study of GANA was conducted with 58 Mexican American families with children with externalizing disorders. The families were randomly assigned to GANA, regular PCIT, or usual care. Families who participated in GANA had significantly better outcomes than families who were given usual care. However, in general, the outcomes for the families who received GANA were not significantly different from those who received PCIT (McCabe & Yeh, 2009).

Multidimensional Treatment Foster Care (MTFC)

MTFC, which was designed by Chamberlain and colleagues at the Oregon Social Learning Center, is a milieu treatment that employs foster parents as agents of change (Fisher & Chamberlain, 2000). Foster parents who participate in MTFC are extensively trained in behavior management. They use a point system that rewards the foster child for engaging in activities that he would normally be expected to do, such as attending classes, and takes away points for breaking the household rules. The foster parent and the child are assisted by a clinical team which includes a Parent Daily Report (PDR) caller, case manager/clinical supervisor, behavior support specialist, youth therapist, family therapist, and consulting psychiatrist. The PDR caller contacts the foster parent daily and they complete a checklist of the problematic behaviors the child engaged in each day. This checklist is given to the clinical supervisor/case manager who coordinates the activities of the rest of the treatment team (Fisher & Chamberlain, 2000).

When conducted with maltreated children, MTFC has proven to be superior to regular foster care at reducing behavior problems and placement breakdown, and improving parenting skills (Chamberlain, 2003; Chamberlain, Price, Leve, Laurent, Landsverk, et al., 2008; Fisher & Chamberlain, 2000; Price, Chamberlain, Landsverk, Reid, Leve, et al., 2008). MTFC has also been implemented in Sweden, the United Kingdom, and Canada, and it is currently being implemented in Norway, Denmark, the Netherlands, and Ireland (TFC Consultants Inc., 2009). Yet effectiveness studies of these MTFC programs have not yet been published. Additionally, while the samples in studies of MTFC programs in the United States have contained minority youth including children who spoke primarily Spanish (Chamberlain et al., 2008), the outcomes of minority youth in comparison to White youth have not been the main focus of the research.

COMPATIBILITY OF TF-CBT, PCIT, AND MTFC WITH CHILDREN FROM IMMIGRANT FAMILIES INVOLVED IN THE CHILD WELFARE SYSTEM

Although TF-CBT, PCIT, and MTFC were not designed for immigrant families, there are many aspects of these treatments that indicate that they could potentially be beneficial for immigrant families in the CWS. For example, not only do these programs have extensive research supporting their efficacy, in contrast with many mental health interventions for immigrant families, these treatments have all been tested with children who have been maltreated and who exhibited symptoms of mental health problems. Additionally, both PCIT and MTFC have been applied to children in foster care. Furthermore, researchers frequently study the application of these interventions with new populations. The results from studies of the implementation of all three programs in other countries may suggest ways in which these programs can be modified for immigrants.

TF-CBT may be especially applicable to immigrant families in the CWS, because children in these families may experience multiple forms of trauma. For example, Hispanic children who immigrate to the United States may witness acts of violence while crossing the border (De Arellano et al., 2005). TF-CBT therapists could help immigrant parents understand the impact these experiences may have on their children, and help the children cope with negative thoughts and feelings related to these events.

Although MTFC has a very different treatment philosophy and style than TF-CBT, it may also be easily adapted to suit the needs of immigrant families with children who have been placed in foster care. Some of the benefits of MTFC are that it has a large treatment team, and that the treatment is provided in a variety of settings: the child's school, community, foster home and biological home. This wrap-around style approach may be valuable for two reasons: First of all, one member of the treatment team could devote his or her time to helping the child deal with acculturative stress while the other members continue to focus on the child's behavior problems. Secondly, if the child is facing discrimination at school and having culturally-related conflicts with both his foster parents and his biological parents, MTFC could address all of these issues.

Finally, while MTFC and TF-CBT have the potential to help immigrant families, there is already some evidence that PCIT is successful with people from non-western cultures. Although GANA was not more successful than regular PCIT, it still led to positive outcomes and was more effective than a no treatment condition.

However, before assuming that these interventions will be successful with immigrant families, additional research, especially on the effectiveness of MTFC with families from non-western cultures, is needed. Additional studies of TF-CBT with children who have been physically abused or neglected are also needed, because immigrant children who are placed in the CWS may be victims of these types of maltreatment. Finally, immigrant parents may be difficult to engage in these programs due to limited English proficiency, possible lack of insurance coverage, and concern about the stigma of mental health treatment (Gudino, Lau, & Hough, 2008).

TREATMENTS THAT HAVE BEEN TESTED WITH BOTH CHILDREN FROM IMMIGRANT FAMILIES AND CHILDREN IN THE CHILD WELFARE SYSTEM

The Incredible Years

The Incredible Years is actually a series of treatment programs. One of the parent-training programs, BASIC, is designed to help parents of infants and children age up to 12 years become more effective disciplinarians and address child behavior problems (Incredible Years, 2008). In 12–14 week sessions, parents watch and discuss videotapes of parent-child interactions. They learn how to play with and praise their children, set limits, and respond to inappropriate behavior (Linares, Montalto, Li, & Oza, 2006; Incredible Years, 2008).

Linares and colleagues (2006) studied the effectiveness of the BASIC program combined with a co-parenting intervention for 128 foster and biological parents of children who were currently in foster care. The co-parenting intervention consisted of one session in which the biological parents met with their child's foster parents and attempted to resolve conflicts about parenting issues. The researchers found that compared to the control group, parents in the intervention group used significantly more positive parenting practices and were significantly better at providing clear expectations after completing treatment.

The effectiveness of the BASIC program has also been studied with a small sample of Korean American mothers and their children. All of the 29 mothers in the study were first-generation immigrants. The program was tested with this population because traditional Korean parenting practices include using harsh discipline and fewer positive interactions with children than standard American parenting practices. The mothers' level of acculturation was measured and included in the analysis.

Following the training, the mothers in the intervention group were more likely to use positive discipline than the mothers in the control group who did not receive any kind of treatment. Furthermore, the researchers found that highly acculturated mothers increased their use of appropriate discipline techniques (time-outs, withdrawal of privileges) while less acculturated mothers decreased their use of harsh discipline (Kim, Cain, & Webster-Stratton, 2008). Although this study had a small sample size and most of the children did not have behavior problems, the results suggest that The Incredible Years may be successfully adapted for immigrant families.

CONCLUSION

The reviews of both evidence-based mental health treatments that have been tested with maltreating families, and family-based mental health treatments for immigrants suggest that the ideal treatment would:

- use engagement strategies to recruit immigrant families;
- address acculturative stress and acculturation conflicts;
- teach parenting techniques;

- address trauma caused by maltreatment and or the immigration experience;
- help parents with their own mental health problems;
- be delivered in immigrant families' native languages; and
- have research support indicating effectiveness with both immigrant families and children who have been maltreated.

As shown in Table 1, none of the treatments in this review have all of the ideal components. Yet, both the interventions for immigrant families and those for maltreated children may be adapted to suit the needs of immigrant families in the CWS. The Incredible Years, MHIP, and TF-CBT may have the most research to support their application to this unique population. The Incredible Years is the only program that has been tested with both families with CWS involvement and immigrants. Also, the treatment used in MHIP is very similar to TF-CBT, which suggests that these types of cognitive behavioral treatments could be effective for immigrant youth in the CWS suffering from depression and PTSD.

However, these youth may vary in the severity of the maltreatment that they have experienced, and in the severity of their psychological disorders. Given the fact that mental health interventions for immigrant families are mostly group-based programs, and are designed for children living with their biological parents, these interventions may be best adapted for families with more mild incidents of maltreatment and for children with less acute mental health problems. Meanwhile, adaptations of individualized treatments such as TF-CBT, PCIT, and MTFC may be better suited for immigrant children with severe psychological problems who have been placed in foster care.

Children from immigrant families in foster care may also need interventions that address cultural conflicts that arise between foster parents who are either uninformed about the child's heritage, or who are at a different level of acculturation than the child. Furthermore, parents in immigrant families may benefit from interventions that, in addition to focusing on intergenerational cultural conflicts, address some of the issues the parents may face such as substance abuse, domestic violence, or difficulties arising from undocumented status. Studies of immigrants have found that they are at risk for developing psychiatric problems and can face many obstacles that prevent them from accessing treatment including concerns about stigma and language barriers (Pumariega, Rothe, & Pumariega, 2005). Researchers and treatment providers seeking to create or adapt mental health interventions for immigrant families should consider the unique needs of all of the family members.

However, researchers and treatment providers should also be aware that parents in immigrant families may face many obstacles to utilization of mental health services (Gudino, Lau, & Hough, 2008). Future research on adapting mental health treatments for immigrant families involved in CWS should focus on whether the intensive engagement strategies used in

TABLE 1 Ideal Components of Mental Health Treatments for Immigrant Families Involved in the Child Welfare System

Program	Uses engagement strategies	Addresses acculturative stress and acculturation conflicts	Addresses parenting difficulties	Addresses trauma caused by maltreatment and/or immigration	Helps parents with their own mental health problems	Offered in immigrant families' native languages	Tested with both immigrant families and children who have been maltreated
Entre Dos Mundos		X				X (Spanish)	
Familias Unidas	X	X	X			X (Spanish)	
Incredible Years			X		X		X
Mental Health for Immigrants Program (MHIP)		X		X	X	X (Spanish)	
Multidimensional Treatment Foster Care (MTFC)			X				
Parent–Child Interaction Therapy (PCIT)	X (GANA)		X			X (Cantonese & Spanish)	
Strengthening of Intergenerational/ Intercultural Ties in Immigrant Chinese American Families (SITICAF)		X	X			X (Mandarin)	
Trauma-Focused Cognitive Behavioral Therapy (TF-CBT)			X	X		X (Spanish)	

Familias Unidas and GANA actually improve parents' treatment engagement and prevent attrition. Further research is needed on whether these strategies can be used with immigrants from non-Spanish speaking cultures. Most of the mental health interventions identified in these reviews were designed or adapted for Hispanics, and research is also needed on the adaptation of mental health treatments for immigrants coming from Asian, African, and European countries.

Children from immigrant families that are involved in the CWS face several risk factors that can be detrimental to their mental health. In order to assist these children and their families, existing mental health treatments designed for immigrant families and those designed for families in the CWS could be modified to address both acculturative stress and the sequelae of maltreatment.

REFERENCES

American Academy of Child and Adolescent Psychiatry. (2005). *Facts for Families: Foster Care.* Retrieved from http://www.aacap.org/cs/root/facts_for_families/foster care.

Barth, R. P., Landsverk, J., Chamberlain, P., Reid, J. B., Rolls, J. A., Hurlburt, M. S. . . . (2005). Parent-training programs in child welfare services: Planning for a more evidence-based approach to serving biological parents. *Research on Social Work Practice, 15*(5), 353–371.

Bolger, K. E., Patterson, C. J., Thompson, W. W., & Kupersmidt, J. B. (1995). Psychosocial adjustment among children experiencing persistent and intermittent economic family hardship. *Child Development, 66*(4), 1107–1129.

Burns, B. J., Phillips, S. D., Wagner, H. R., Barth, R. P., Kolko, D. J., Campbell, Y. . . . (2004). Mental health need and access to mental health services by youths involved with child welfare: A national survey. *Journal of the American Academy of Child and Adolescent Psychiatry, 43*(8), 960–970.

Chaffin, M., Silovsky, J. F., Funderburk, B., Valle, L. A., Brestan, E. V., Balachova, T. . . . (2004). Parent-child interaction therapy with physically abusive parents: Efficacy for reducing future abuse reports. *Journal of Consulting and Clinical Psychology, 72*(3), 500–510.

Chahine, Z., & Van Straaten, J. (2005). Serving immigrant families and children in New York City's child welfare system. *Child Welfare, 84*(5), 713–723.

Chamberlain, P. (2003). The Oregon multidimensional treatment foster care model: Features, outcomes, and progress in dissemination. *Cognitive and Behavioral Practice, 10*(303–312).

Chamberlain, P., Price, J., Leve, L. D., Laurent, H., Landsverk, J., & Reid, J. B. (2008). Prevention of behavior problems for children in foster care: Outcomes and mediation effects. *Prevention Science, 9*, 17–27.

Clausen, J. M., Landsverk, J., Ganger, W., Chadwick, D., & Litronik, A. (1998). Mental health problems of children in foster care. *Journal of Child and Family Studies, 7*(3), 283–296.

Cohen, J. A., Mannarino, A. P., Murray, L. K., & Igelman, R. (2006). Psychosocial interventions for maltreated and violence-exposed children. *Journal of Social Issues, 62*(4), 737–766.

Coohey, C. (1996). Child maltreatment: Testing the social isolation hypothesis. *Child Abuse & Neglect, 20*(3), 241–254.

De Arellano, M. A. (2009, January). *Culturally-modified trauma-focused cognitive behavior therapy*. Presentation at the 23rd Annual San Diego International Conference on Child and Family Maltreatment, San Diego, CA.

De Arellano, M. A., Ko, S. J., Danielson, C. K. & Sprague, C. M. (2008). *Trauma-informed interventions: Clinical and research evidence and culture-specific information project*. Durham, NC: National Center for Child Traumatic Stress.

De Arellano, M. A., Waldrop, A. E., Deblinger, E., Cohen, J. A., & Mannarino, A. P. (2005). Community outreach program for child victims of traumatic events: A community–based project for underserved populations. *Behavior Modification, 29*(1), 130–155.

Dettlaff, A. J., Earner, I., & Phillips, S. D. (2009). Hispanic children of immigrants in the child welfare system: Prevalence, characteristics and risk. *Children and Youth Services Review, 31*, 775–783.

Fisher, P. A., & Chamberlain, P. (2000). Multidimensional treatment foster care: A program for intensive parenting, family support, and skill building. *Journal of Emotional and Behavioral Disorders, 8*(3), 155–164.

Fortuny, K. Capps, R., Simms, M., & Chaudry, A. (2009). Children of immigrants: National and state characteristics. Washington, DC: Urban Institute.

Garland, A. F., Landsverk, J., Hough, R. L., & Ellis–MacLeod, E. (1996). Type of maltreatment as a predictor of mental health service use for children in foster care. *Child Abuse & Neglect, 20*(8), 675–688.

Gudino, O. G., Lau, A. S., & Hough, R. (2008). Immigrant status, mental health need and mental health utilization among high-risk Hispanic and Asian Pacific Islander youth. *Child Youth Care Forum, 37*, 139–152.

Herschell, A. D., Calzada, E. J., Eyberg, S. M., & McNeil, C. B. (2002). Parent–child interaction therapy: New directions in research. *Cognitive and Behavioral Practice, 9*, 9–16.

Incredible Years. (2008). *Incredible years parent training programs 2008*. Retrieved from http://www.incredibleyears.com/program/parent.asp

Kataoka, S. H., Stein, B. D., Jaycox, L. H., Wong, M., Escudero, P., Tu, W. . . . (2003). A school–based mental health program for traumatized Hispanic immigrant children. *Journal of the American Academy of Child and Adolescent Psychiatry, 42*(3), 311–317.

Kerker, B. D., & Dore, M. M. (2006). Mental health needs and treatment of foster youth: Barriers and opportunities. *American Journal of Orthopsychiatry, 76*(1), 138–147.

Kim, E., Cain, K., & Webster-Stratton, C. (2008). The preliminary effect of a parenting program to Korean American mothers: A randomized controlled trial. *International Journal of Nursing Studies, 45*(9), 1261–1273.

Lau, A. S., & Weisz, J. R. (2003). Reported maltreatment among clinic-referred children: Implications for presenting problems, treatment attrition, and long-term outcomes. *Journal of the American Academy of Child and Adolescent Psychiatry, 42*(11), 1327–1334.

Leung, C., Tsang, S., Heung, K., & Yiu, I. (2009). Effectiveness of parent–child interaction therapy among Chinese families. *Research on Social Work Practice, 19*(3), 304–313.

Linares, L. O., Montalto, D., Li, M., & Oza, V. S. (2006). A promising parenting intervention in foster care. *Journal of Consulting and Clinical Psychology, 74*(1), 32–41.

Matos, M., Torres, R., Santiago, R., Jurado, M., & Rodriguez, I. (2006). Adaptation of parent–child interaction therapy for Puerto Rican families: A preliminary study. *Family Process, 45*(2), 205–222.

McCabe, K. M., & Yeh, M. (2009). Parent–child interaction therapy for Mexican American families: A randomized clinical trial. *Journal of Clinical Child and Adolescent Psychology, 38*(5), 753–759.

McCabe, K. M., Yeh, M., Garland, A. F., Lau, A. S., & Chavez, G. (2005). The GANA program: A tailoring approach to adapting parent–child interaction therapy for Mexican Americans. *Education and Treatment of Children, 28*(2), 111–129.

Murray, L. K., Cohen, J. A., Ellis, B. H., & Mannarino, A. P. (2008). Cognitive behavior therapy for symptoms of trauma and traumatic grief in refugee youth. *Child and Adolescent Psychiatric Clinics of North America, 17*, 585–604.

National Child Traumatic Stress Network. (2005). Mental health interventions for refugee children in resettlement. Retrieved from http://nctsn.org/nctsn_assets/pdfs/promising_practices/MH_Interventions_for_Refugee_Children.pdf

Pantin, H., Coatsworth, J. D., Feaster, D. J., Newman, F. L., Briones, E., Prado, G. . . . (2003). Familias Unidas: The efficacy of an intervention to promote parental investment in Hispanic immigrant families. *Prevention Science, 4*(3), 189–201.

Portes, A., & Rumbaut, R. G. (2001). *Legacies: The story of the immigrant second generation*. Berkeley, CA: University of California Press.

Price, J., Chamberlain, P., Landsverk, J., Reid, J. B., Leve, L. D., & Laurent, H. (2008). Effects of a foster parent training intervention on placement changes of children in foster care. *Child Maltreatment, 13*(1), 64–75.

Pumariega, A. J., Rothe, E., & Pumariega, J. B. (2005). Mental health of immigrants and refugees. *Community Mental Health Journal, 41*(5), 581–597.

Raj, A., & Sliverman, J. (2002). Violence against women: The role of culture, context and legal immigrant status on intimate partner violence. *Violence Against Women, 8*, 367–398.

Rousseau, C., Benoit, M., Gauthier, M. F., Lacroix, L., Alain, N., Rojas, M. V. . . . (2007). Classroom drama therapy program for immigrant and refugee adolescents: A pilot study. *Clinical Child Psychology and Psychiatry, 12*, 451–465.

Segal, U. A., & Mayadas, N. S. (2005). Assessment of issues facing immigrant and refugee families. *Child Welfare, 84*(5), 563–583.

Shipman, K., & Taussig, H. (2009). Mental health treatment of child abuse and neglect: The promise of evidence–based practice. *Pediatric Clinics of North America, 56*, 417–428.

Sluzki, C. E. (1979). Migration and family conflict. *Family Process, 18*(4), 379–390.

Smokowski, P. R., & Bacallao, M. (2009). Entre Dos Mundos/Between two worlds: Youth violence prevention for acculturating Hispanic families. *Research on Social Work Practice, 19*(2), 165–178.

Stein, B. D., Kataoka, S., Jaycox, L., Steiger, E. M., Wong, M., Fink, A. . . . (2003). The mental health for immigrants program: Program design and participatory research in the real world. In *Handbook of School Mental Health*, M. D. Weist, S. W. Evans, and N. A. Lever (eds.) New York, NY: Springer, 179–190.

Tapia, M. I., Schwartz, S. J., Lopez, B., & Pantin, H. (2006). Parent–centered intervention: A practical approach for preventing drug abuse in Hispanic adolescents. *Research on Social Work Practice, 16*(2), 6–165.

TFC Consultants, Inc. (2009). *MTFC Program Certification*. Retrieved from http://www.mtfc.com/currentsites.html

Timmer, S. G., Urquiza, A. J., Herschell, A. D., McGrath, J. M., Zebell, N. M., Porter, A. L. . . . (2006). Parent–child interaction therapy: Application of an empirically supported treatment to maltreated children in foster care. *Child Welfare, 85*(6), 919–939.

Timmer, S. G., Urquiza, A. J., & Zebell, N. (2006). Challenging foster caregiver–maltreated child relationships: The effectiveness of parent–child interaction therapy. *Children and Youth Services Review, 28*(1), 1–19.

Timmer, S. G., Urquiza, A. J., Zebell, N. M., & McGrath, J. M. (2005). Parent–child interaction therapy: Application to maltreating parent–child dyads. *Child Abuse & Neglect, 29*, 825–842.

Vericker, T., Kuehn, D., & Capps, R. (2007). *Foster care placement settings and permanency planning: Patterns by child generation and ethnicity*. Washington, DC: Urban Institute.

Ying, Y. (1999). Strengthening intergenerational/intercultural ties in migrant families: A new intervention for parents. *Journal of Community Psychology, 27*(1), 89–96.

Ying, Y., & Han, M. (2007). The longitudinal effect of intergenerational gap in acculturation on conflict and mental health in Southeast Asian American adolescents. *American Journal of Orthopsychiatry, 77*(1), 61–66.

Child Welfare and Immigration in New Mexico: Challenges, Achievements, and the Future

MEGAN FINNO

and

MARYELLEN BEARZI

Immigration—specifically, the migration of families between the United States and the United Mexican States—claims a significant piece of New Mexico's history. Recently national attention has focused on the impact on families of this migration and the resulting outcomes This article outlines the immigration issues experienced by families touching the New Mexico child welfare system, including the challenges created in the intersection of child welfare and migration from the perspective of a border state; the application of national recommendations for child welfare practice and achievements; and ongoing work aimed at enhancing response and intervention with immigrant families. This article also highlights the policies adopted and the partnerships involving child protection agencies and advocates on both sides of the New Mexico/Mexico border that have forged to meet the needs of the children and families.

Immigration, and more specifically, the migration of families between the United States and the United Mexican States (Mexico), claims a significant piece of New Mexico's history. The impact and outcomes on families and children resulting from this migration have begun receiving national attention in recent years. In 2006, university and non-profit experts initiated a discussion among a network of leaders in the fields of social welfare and immigration that resulted in a published set of recommendations for serving immigrant families in child welfare (Dettlaff, Vidal de Haymes, Velazquez, Mindell & Bruce, 2009; Velasquez, Vidal de Haymes, & Mindell, 2006).

The newly formalized Migration and Child Welfare National Network, has drawn attention to the enormity of the obstacles and stressors faced by immigrant families and the child welfare systems that respond to them. Recommendations for best practice reflect multiple factors and various facets of the child welfare system; address research, data collection, policy and training issues; and the ethical issues that may arise in the process (Dettlaff, Vidal de Haymes, Velazquez, Mindell, & Bruce, 2009).

This article outlines immigration issues experienced in the New Mexico child welfare system, including the ongoing challenges identified in the intersection of child welfare and migration from the perspective of a border state; the application of national recommendations for child welfare practice in the state and achievements; and ongoing goals for enhancing response and intervention with immigrant families. This article also highlights the policies adopted and the partnerships that have forged in the past year to meet the needs of these children and families, through support from child protection agencies and advocates on both sides of the New Mexico/Mexico border.

BACKGROUND

In the United States, more than 30% of the immigrant population is undocumented (Passel, 2006). It is estimated that undocumented immigrants number 11.9 million nationwide, approximately 4% of the total population (Passel & Cohn, 2009). Approximately 75% (76%) of the nation's undocumented population are from Latin America (Passel & Cohn, 2009; Capps & Passell, 2004; U.S. Census Bureau, 2006). Mexico is the source of the largest numbers, accounting for 59% of the undocumented immigrants in the United States (Passel & Cohn, 2009).

Nationally, 33% of children of undocumented parents and 20% of adult undocumented immigrants live in poverty (Passel & Cohn, 2009). More than one in ten U.S. families with children is a mixed immigration status family (i.e., families with at least one non-citizen parent and one child who is a citizen) (Passel, 2006). In 2008, an estimated 5.5 million children (more than 7% of all children living in the United States) had undocumented parents (Passel & Cohn, 2009). Approximately 75% of these children, or 4 million, were U.S.-born citizens (Passel & Cohn, 2009).

Most recent figures indicate that unauthorized immigrants living in the United States are more geographically dispersed than in the past (Passel & Cohn, 2009). However, unauthorized Mexican immigrants have been found to be somewhat more concentrated than all other undocumented immigrants, accounting for high proportions of the undocumented immigrant population in a few states (Passel & Cohn, 2009).

Immigration in New Mexico

New Mexico is crouched between the more highly populated states of Texas and Arizona, sharing its southern border with Mexico's northern border. A large state geographically, New Mexico's population hovers approximately 2 million residents who are mostly concentrated in a few high population areas. Immigrants in New Mexico, not unlike other areas of the country, have been seen in large metro areas of the state, such as Albuquerque in the central section, and Las Cruces in the south (Passel & Cohn, 2009). However, in recent years, smaller communities around Santa Fe in northern New Mexico and eastern New Mexico have also been impacted by a strong immigrant presence.

New Mexico's demographic is reflective of a dynamic typical in border areas across the region where transnational migration is prevalent. Migration, once perceived as a singular, directed movement involving a sending state and a receiving state, is seen in a transnational context as an ongoing movement between two or more countries. More and more migrants to the United States have developed strong transnational ties to more than one home country, manifested in strong interconnectivity among peoples, governments, and organizations, and often creating duality in economic, cultural, social and political activities (Basch, Glick-Schiller, & Szanton-Blanc, 1994). The prevalence of transnationalism is widespread in the border area of New Mexico, as many families split by the U.S.-Mexico border travel back and forth on a regular basis for shopping, education, medical care, and to visit with family and friends.

Immigration is a contested issue in New Mexico, containing areas that support a pro-immigrant stance and others that have adopted local policies of intolerance. The city of Santa Fe is designated a "sanctuary city" by local government. Other communities in the state have developed informal policies of intolerance of undocumented immigrants, and some local law enforcement agencies have reportedly collaborated in arrest and detainment activities with immigration enforcement agencies along the border.[1] However, in 2009, New Mexico became the twenty-third state to ban racial profiling (New Mexico Legislature, 2009). This new law is expected to impact immigrant communities that are routinely questioned about immigration status by local law enforcement agencies. Local agencies and grassroots organizations are currently working in their respective communities to ensure that local police agencies comply with this legislation.

New Mexico is not a traditional high destination state for immigrants to the United States, nor is it one of the 22 states that experienced the most rapid growth in immigration during the 1990s (Capps & Fortuny, 2006). Nevertheless, New Mexico's immigrant population has grown significantly in the past decade, nearly on par with current trends nationwide (U.S. Census Bureau, 2006). In New Mexico, in 2008, there were an estimated 80,000 undocumented immigrants (4% of state population), up from 55,000 in 2000 (Passel & Cohn, 2009). New Mexico is one of three states in which 90% of the undocumented population has their origins in Mexico (Passel & Cohn, 2009).

These figures are significant because Mexicans are more likely than other undocumented immigrants to have children (Passel & Cohn, 2009). They are also less educated and have lower incomes than other undocumented immigrants (Passel & Cohn, 2009). In New Mexico, it is estimated that at least 20% of children in New Mexico are children of immigrants (Capps & Fortuny, 2006). An estimated 85% of children with immigrant parents in New Mexico have at least one parent from Latin America, most of whose origins are in Mexico (New Mexico Voices for Children, 2007; Passel & Cohn, 2009).

Challenges to Immigrants in New Mexico

The challenges faced by immigrant families in New Mexico are not few. In New Mexico, 34% of children in immigrant families live in a linguistically isolated household, and approximately 17% of immigrant children live in families in which their parents have a less than ninth-grade education (New Mexico Voices for Children, 2007). Also, 37% of immigrant children live below the poverty threshold, compared with 24% of children in U.S.-born families (New Mexico Voices for Children, 2007). In addition, 71% of children live in low-income families, versus 50% of children in US born families in the state (New Mexico Voices for Children, 2007).

In the Albuquerque metro area and surrounding areas of northern New Mexico, it is estimated that, currently, 24% to 29% of children live in immigrant families (Annie E. Casey, 2009), higher than the state average. These areas also represent larger concentrations of child welfare cases involving immigrant families than other more rural parts of the state (Finno, Reyes, Espinoza Rodriguez, & Gallardo Robles, 2010). Up to 44% of children are estimated to be living in immigrant families in areas on the border, such as the border town of Deming, New Mexico (Annie E. Casey, 2009). While the number of immigrant children and families in the New Mexico child welfare system is relatively small, the associated risks and complexity of these cases, combined with the growth of the immigrant population in New Mexico, demonstrates the need for child welfare to continue examining and addressing the needs of this population.

CHILD WELFARE AND IMMIGRATION

Risks and Vulnerabilities

The risks for involvement in the child welfare system associated with the immigration experience in New Mexico are comparable to the issues immigrants face in mid to large urban areas across the country, and are widely documented (Capps, Fix, Ost, Reardon-Anderson, & Passel, 2004; Partida, 1996; Pine & Drachman, 2005; Smart & Smart, 1995; Padilla & Perez, 2003; Hovey, 2000; Thoman & Suris, 2004). Current data support the assertion that undocumented immigrants from Latin American countries are primarily young, poor, have little formal education, and speak little to no English (Passel & Cohn, 2009). The driving force in the decision to migrate is most often based on financial necessity or dangerous political situations in the country of origin (Partida, 1996). Many immigrants experience robbery, violence, physical persecution, and sexual assault in the process of immigration (Solis, 2003). Families often migrate in stages, which results in children being separated from their parents and other family members for extended periods of time (Partida, 1996; Pine & Drachman, 2005). The stress, trauma and loss associated with this initial transition period can result in issues such as depression, anxiety and post-traumatic stress disorder (Smart & Smart, 1995).

Once arrived to the United States, immigrants are increasingly vulnerable due to language barriers, difficulty in obtaining employment, unfamiliar customs, loss of support systems, ongoing threats of violence or deportation, and exposure to social discrimination and prejudice (Hancock, 2005; Padilla & Perez, 2003; Solis, 2003; Smart & Smart, 1995). The loss of support and the increased stress in navigating new systems have been associated with psychological problems such as depression, anxiety and alcoholism (Leon & Dziegielewski, 1999). Undocumented immigrants are less likely to access needed resources or services due to a sense of caution or mistrust in relationships and fear of deportation (Pine & Drachman, 2005; Smart & Smart, 1995). Furthermore, many immigrants have cultural norms that differ from those in the United States, in the areas of child rearing, discipline, supervision and medical treatment. In some child welfare agencies, cultural differences in parenting styles have been viewed as negligence (Olayo Mendez, 2006; Zielewski, Malm, & Geen, 2006).

Acculturation—or the process of change experienced by immigrants with exposure to a new culture—often causes significant stress to immigrants, particularly to those whose host cultures are distinct in ethnicity, religion, and language (Padilla & Perez, 2003). Extensive research on acculturative stress has linked this process to anxiety, depression, substance abuse, declining health and physical functioning, and diminished coping skills in adults and adolescents (Alderete, Vega, Kolody, & Aguilar-Gaxiola, 1999; Finch, Frank, & Vega, 2004; Miranda & Matheny, 2000; Thoman & Suris, 2004). The process of acculturation has been found to increase tensions and conflict between children and parents as values change, and contributes to parental loss of control (Fontes, 2002). Acculturative stress has also shown to place significant stress on marital relationships as traditional gender roles change, and increase the risk of domestic violence in the home (Coltrane, Park & Adams, 2004; Cunradi, Caetano, & Shafer, 2002).

Despite high levels of poverty, physical and emotional vulnerability, and increased risk of mental health issues and family conflict, immigrant families possess a key protective factor that may contribute to under-involvement in the child welfare system. Children of immigrants have been found to be relatively less likely than their counterparts to live in a single parent household in the United States, potentially lowering their risk of involvement with the child welfare system (Vericker, Kuehn, & Capps, 2007).

The Children, Youth, and Families Department Protective Services Division (PSD)

The Children, Youth, and Families Department Protective Services Division (PSD) is the state public child welfare agency in New Mexico. Despite the heightened risks and vulnerabilities associated with undocumented im-migration, PSD estimates that the number of undocumented children and children of immigrants in PSD custody is comparatively lower than anecdotal reports from other states (Finno, Reyes, Espinoza Rodriguez, & Gallardo Robles, 2010). The number of undocumented children steadily account for approximately 1% to 2% of the approximately 2,000 children in custody across the state (Finno et al., 2010). Although it has historically been a challenge to track citizenship status of parents involved in the child welfare system in New Mexico, current estimations indicate that approximately 6% of children in custody are immigrants or children of immigrants (Finno et al., 2010). Most immigrant families, more than 90%, who come to the attention of PSD, have their origins in Mexico (Finno et al., 2010).

In the past, the PSD involvement with immigrant families was concen-trated in the southern border region of the state and in the Albuquerque metro area. However, in recent years, the shifting population had affected rural offices across the state with little previous experience with immigra-tion (Finno et al., 2010). These cases have become more widespread and complex, involving families with varying legal statuses residing in multiple nation states, and demanding more resources to adequately and effectively serve them.

PSD PRACTICE AND INTERVENTION

PSD "believes in the strengths and resiliency of all families in New Mexico and advocates to enhance their safety and well-being ... PSD serves and supports children and families in a responsive, community-based system of care that is client-centered, family-focused and culturally competent" (New Mexico Children, Youth, and Families Department, 2009). Central among the core principles of PSD is the declaration that culturally competent services are delivered without regard to race, ethnicity, religion, national origin, gender, sexual orientation, or disability. PSD serves children and families in New Mexico regardless of national origin or immigration status (New Mexico Children, Youth, and Families Department, 2009). Though an undocumented legal status impedes access to federal funds for service, New Mexico has committed to ensuring equitable quality service for all residents regardless of legal status using state funding. PSD is not required to share confidential information with federal immigration authorities. PSD is bound by and upholds confidentiality law, and PSD considers immigration status to be confidential information.

Expectations placed upon New Mexico child welfare workers are high as best practices and standards for service in working with immigrant families are becoming more clearly defined (Lincroft, Resner, Leung, & Bussiere, 2006). Several best practice models exist that define critical steps in effectively serving immigrant families in any child welfare system (Georgia Department of Human Resources, 2009; University of New Mexico Corinne Wolfe Children's Law Center, 2007; Earner, 2005, 2007; New York City Administration for Children's Services, 2005; Pine & Drachman, 2005; Vidal de Haymes, 2005; Fong, 2004). Initial and ongoing training in child welfare practice in New Mexico has begun to emphasize many of these special considerations for working with immigrant families.

A family's legal status contributes to the structuring of the immigration experience and creates challenges to family well-being; thus this status is a primary factor to consider in assessing and determining appropriate interventions by the child welfare system (Lincroft Resner, Leung, & Bussiere, 2006). PSD investigators are most often the immigrant family's first point of contact with the agency. Some initial inquiries made in interviewing parents when children come into custody serve to determine each family member's legal status in the United States. These frontline staff have been trained to frame questions about legal status delicately, to inform families that PSD does not release information regarding legal status to any law enforcement entity, unless that information is subpoenaed by law enforcement in court (State of New Mexico, 2009b). They are trained to clarify PSD's reason for inquiry; to comply with consular notification requirements; to provide families with referrals for legal assistance to their country of origin's foreign consulate; and to determine eligibility for federally funded resources and services (State of New Mexico, 2009b). PSD's Title IV-E unit specializes in determining and verifying eligibility for federal IV-E and other benefits in the inception of and throughout a case. This unit also assists in determining legal status for parents and children in custody, and participates in a new process for streamlining and tracking all cases involving non-U.S. citizen children and/or parents in one centralized database.

In addition, PSD has increased emphasis in practice on determining and providing for the language needs of each family member involved in a case. Standardized forms have been reviewed and translated into Spanish through a contracted certified translation agency, and the need for additional translations in other languages is reviewed centrally on an ongoing basis. PSD has issued internal guidelines for ensuring language needs are met, which mandate that competent interpretation services be arranged for all clients that prefer them. These guidelines specify that it is allowable to utilize an adult family member, volunteer or other professional as an interpreter in a case as long as their qualifications and proficiency can be verified. PSD also employs many personnel who are proficient in Spanish, many of whom speak Spanish at home, and have been designated to serve as interpreters for clients in field offices when their schedules allow. PSD has contracted with a service provider statewide for phone interpretation services should no interpreter be available in person. This system has served to maximize resources with minimal budget to ensure that families have access to quality language assistance.

Apart from legal status and language needs, there are several other special factors that require attention in child welfare intervention with immigrant families and have been outlined in literature in recent years (Borelli, K., Earner, I., & Lincroft, L., 2008; Dettlaff & Rycraft, 2006; Earner, 2007; Fong, 2004). Positive outcomes require a child welfare workforce that understands the issues, laws and needs pertaining to immigrant families (Dettlaff et al., 2009). Towards this end, over the past year, PSD has conducted all-staff trainings on working with immigrants, and has designated employees and realigned resources to create in-house expertise in immigration issues in order to: provide coaching and assistance in staffing complicated cases; attend immigration related appointments with clients and workers; guide workers and clients through various immigration applications; and locate interpreter services and translate key documents for the agency. New Mexico's challenges and achievements in practice with immigrant families are detailed in the sections to follow.

Challenges to Practice in New Mexico

PSD faces a variety of challenges in working with immigrant families, some that are similar to those challenges documented by the Migration and Child Welfare National Network, and others that are particularly unique to New Mexico (Dettlaff et al., 2009; Lincroft et al., 2006). Cross-systems collaboration is an area of great challenge albeit a necessity for PSD. As a border state, New Mexico relies on international, federal, state, and local partners in coordinating efforts to serve immigrants seamlessly across systems. A recent challenge related to cross system collaboration pertains to the impact of immigration raids and enforcement activities on families (Capps, Castaneda, Chaudry & Santos, 2007; Chaudry, Capps, Pedroza, Castaneda, Santos, & Scott, 2009). Immigration raids and enforcement activities were documented in New Mexico in 2007 and 2008, although PSD was not notified to respond nor have any children come into custody as a direct result of these activities (State of New Mexico, 2008). PSD was not routinely informed of enforcement operations before they happened. It is expected that relatives, neighbors, friends, and community agencies absorbed the responsibility of caring for children left without parents, as was documented in other areas of the country (Capps et al., 2007). This lack of initial involvement by PSD to ensure the safety and well-being of children who were separated from their parents may place them at an additional risk of later entering into the system. The lasting impact of these enforcement activities has been documented to be manifested in ongoing family separation, employment, housing and food hardship, and increased child fear and anxiety (Chaudry et al., 2009). Though humanitarian guidelines have reportedly been implemented by Immigration and Customs Enforcement (ICE) to minimize the separation of children from their families in workforce raids, and enforcement operations have been narrowed to focus on immigrants who have committed serious crimes, PSD remains witness to ICE's local practices that continue to separate families and children and burden the child welfare system.[2]

Additionally, several common policy issues are related to cross-system collaborations in transnational cases in New Mexico that result in significant delays in permanency. One significant problem is that when a parent is located in another country, PSD has difficulty serving the parent with notice of proceedings and relevant court documents. There have been questions around the sufficiency of serving the foreign consulate with notice in lieu of the parent respondent, and other questions regarding the requirement for publication on a parent living in another country.

One issue that creates barriers to permanency arises in attempts to effectively involve the parent residing out of country in case planning and attending court hearings concerning their child. In scarce circumstances, PSD has been able to petition and obtain day passes from Customs and Border Patrol (CBP) for parents to appear in court. If a parent has had any history with criminal or immigration proceedings in the United States, this petition is not an option. While passes are sometimes granted, the lengthy process involved in obtaining the pass often creates the need to delay court proceedings, resulting in delays in achieving permanency. In transnational cases, PSD has had intermittent success in relying on foreign child welfare agencies to provide services identified in PSD court mandated case plans. However, many court plans implemented in foreign countries have not been completed due to systematic differences in services and policies, and in many cases a parent's lack of access to adequate behavioral health, parenting, and substance abuse services in another country.

New Mexico's situation on the border intensifies many issues related to cross-system collaboration and permanency planning. A common border phenomenon posing a challenge to PSD occurs when U.S. citizens cross the border to Mexico and give birth there. Mexico's system for birth registry differs from the U.S. system in that hospitals in Mexico do not register and create birth certificates when children are born. The responsibility to register a birth and create a birth certificate with Mexico's civil registry falls on the parent subsequent to the birth. In several PSD cases, child births were not registered by parents in Mexico, and on return to the United States, parents did not register the child or adjust status with U.S. authorities, making a birth record non-existent. When these children come into PSD custody, it is known that they should derive U.S. citizenship through their parents, but if no birth record exists, it cannot be proven. Some cases of this nature have resulted in years of delay in finalizing adoptions and gaining access to federal funds for these children. PSD has had to work creatively with other government agencies to create permanency depending on individual circumstances. Creative solutions have included the creation of a New Mexico birth certificate court-ordered by a district judge, obtaining a foreign passport or border entry information through the U.S. Department of State, and DNA tests-court ordered and conducted for parents and children to prove citizenship.

Occasionally, PSD receives custody of U.S. citizen children who have been taken into custody in border cities in Mexico and returned to New Mexico when they are determined to have been abandoned, kidnapped, or abused by parents who had taken them across the border. Other cases involve children who come into custody in New Mexico for abuse or neglect while in the care of friends or family after their parents' deportation. Other times children come into custody after living with caregivers whose parents believe that the children are "better off" living and attending school in New Mexico while visiting with parents across the border on holidays and weekends. Cases become extremely complicated when part of a family lives in a border town in Mexico, and some members live, attend school, and work on the U.S. side of the border during the day or during part of the week. PSD is limited in options for responding to the needs of these families because workers may not travel to Mexico to complete investigations and supervise visits between parents and children. Likewise, foster parents are not permitted to take foster children across the border to run errands, as PSD has no jurisdiction over a child once they have crossed the border to Mexico.

Another area of contention in case planning with parents in Mexico is in the ability to carry out visitation mandates between parents and children. Local offices in border towns with Mexico have worked diligently to over-come this obstacle and have had intermittent success in facilitating parent-child visits at the Port of Entry building in Columbus, NM, a U.S. federal building. PSD has received permission from local CBP officials to conduct visits and depositions in the public lobby area of the building. However, no clear policy exists within the Department of Homeland Security that would establish protocol and guidelines on visitation of this sort.

In addition to a variety of logical challenges, PSD faces some serious ethical dilemmas in the decision-making process in transnational cases. A great predicament revolves around placement decisions for children and how best interest is defined and determined in these cases. In general, when foreign national children enter into custody due to separation from their parents, the primary goal is to reunify them with their parents and maintain family unity, as long as no significant safety risks are identified. However, circumstances become complicated when the definition of best interest is expanded to consider a child's well-being in terms of language, culture, education, opportunity, and legal permanency. For example, in cases in which children are U.S. citizens, having been born and lived in the United States their entire lives, reunifying them with one or both parents may involve moving them to a country and culture unknown to them, separating them from all known sources of strength and support. In other cases involving abuse and neglect, reunification of children with undocumented parents residing in the United States may pose a risk to child well-being and stability if the parent does not have legal permanency in the United States. In such cases, children could potentially be set up for additional trauma due to separation from parents and loss of a primary caregiver if the undocumented parent is detained and/or deported. PSD aims to prevent personal value judgments and decisions made from a biased cultural lens from determining outcomes in transnational cases by maintaining the principle of family unity as a primary factor in defining best interest.

ACHIEVEMENTS IN NEW MEXICO

PSD has quickly evolved to address many of the aforementioned challenges and growing needs of the immigrant population in the child welfare system in New Mexico. Some offices around the state, mostly in the border region, have been informally working with undocumented and mixed status families for years, and have ensured quality practices by maintaining the principle of family unity at the forefront of their decision-making process. In other rural areas of the state, child welfare offices are just beginning to see their first cases with immigrants. PSD is diligently evaluating recommendations and adapting local practices into workable policies and procedures and implementing them around the state.[3]

As part of a multi-pronged approach to addressing issues and needs of immigrant families in the child welfare system, New Mexico has introduced and revised key policies related to immigration mandates in PSD's regulations, currently pending publication. Additionally, New Mexico has recently formalized previously informal relationships with representatives from critical partnering agencies such as the Consulate General of Mexico in El Paso (presiding over the nine southern New Mexico counties), the

Consulate of Mexico in Albuquerque (with jurisdiction over the remaining 24 counties), and child protection partners in Mexico, the *Procuraduria para la Defensa del Menor, la Mujer y la Familia* (PDMMF, Office for the Defense of Children, Women and Families), a division of the *Desarrollo Integral de La Familia* (DIF). PSD is using this formal agreement as a foundation for a strong program for working with immigrants from all countries.

Memorandum of Understanding

The *"Memorandum of Understanding between the Consulate General of Mexico in El Paso, the Consulate of Mexico in Albuquerque, and PSD regarding consular functions in custody proceedings involving Mexican minors as well as mutual collaboration"* (herein referred to as MOU) was signed on March 5, 2009, after over a year of negotiations. This agreement served as a catalyst around which PSD has built infrastructure and standards for working with all immigrant families. This MOU is unique in that it defines multiple areas of collaborative policies and protocols, casework, outreach activities and a working relationship to address partnerships as future needs dictate. Key provisions of the MOU include the determination of Mexican nationality, terms for consular notification and access, interviewing of a Mexican minor, and various areas for mutual collaboration.

According to the MOU, and in concordance with the Mexican Constitution, a "Mexican national" is any person who was born in Mexico or elsewhere of at least one Mexican national parent, regardless of immigration status in the United States. PSD's policy regarding foreign national children, with its basis in international law, the Vienna Convention on Consular Relations of 1967, mandates that when given custody of a foreign national child, PSD will notify the foreign consulate in writing without delay after obtaining custody. PSD recently expanded procedure to include notice to a central PSD immigration liaison when PSD receives custody of a U.S. citizen child with at least one parent who is a foreign national, to determine whether it is in the child's best interest to notify the foreign consulate pertaining to the parent's national origin. PSD's policy on consular notification has been further enhanced to mandate notification when PSD receives custody of a Mexican citizen child or of a U.S. citizen who has at least one parent who is a Mexican citizen. The MOU specifies that if PSD is unaware of a child's Mexican nationality and learns at a later time that a child is a Mexican national, the notification will be forwarded to the Consulate on discovery of Mexican nationality. It further establishes that allowable case information will be shared with the Mexican Consulate for the purposes of service and intervention. In response to this strengthened partnership, the New Mexico Children's Code statute was revised in 2009 to give access to and share confidential case related information with foreign consulates for the purpose of service (New Mexico Children's Code, 1978).

Additionally, the MOU has established procedures for working together with DIF in locating parents and family members of Mexican minors who come into PSD's custody and require placements. It develops a path for obtaining relevant documents, such as birth certificates, medical records and other necessary information to assist in locating relatives and facilitating prompt resolution of cases involving Mexican minors in PSD custody. It establishes a method to formally request investigation of potential placements in Mexico for Mexican minors in PSD custody, including socioeconomic home studies, psychological evaluations, substance abuse evaluations, and the monitoring of placements in Mexico. It provides for collaboration on cases in which Mexican national parents are residing in Mexico and wish to participate in court hearings, treatment plans, and visitation.

The MOU also defines the process for collaboration in the repatriation of Mexican minors in appropriate circumstances to parents or relatives in Mexico. It defines collaboration where a parent may have crossed the border with the intention of evading local authorities and laws involving child abuse. It also provides for cross-agency collaboration on cases in which Mexican parents have children who are born in a U.S. hospital in New Mexico or receive medical care in New Mexico. The MOU pronounces consular support and assistance in providing documentation for immigration relief options, such as Special Immigrant Juvenile status, or the U-visas or T-visas for victims of domestic violence, trafficking or other severe crimes, available to eligible Mexican nationals involved with PSD.

Finally, the MOU encourages joint participation in outreach activities, such as mobile consulates and information sessions with immigrant-serving providers and communities. This enhanced case collaboration has lead to the Mexican Consulate's inclusion in some PSD court hearings, facilitated family centered meetings, and other realms of service planning.

Special Immigrant Juvenile Status (SIJS)

SIJS is an immigration status created by federal law that provides a basis for eligible foreign national children in PSD custody to become lawful permanent residents of the United States. In 2009, the New Mexico Children's Code statute added a section on SIJS and defined roles and timeframes for PSD, attorneys, and the courts in applying for and obtaining SIJS for children in care (New Mexico Children's Code, 1978). Simultaneously, PSD revised policy (pending publication), created new procedures and developed a resource and instruction guide for staff involved in this process of identifying and filing for eligible children (State of New Mexico, 2009a).

This change has been significant as it has created greater assurance that any child eligible for SIJS will be identified and has achieved greater precision and efficiency in the application process. PSD's experience has demonstrated that if children eligible for SIJS are not identified in a timely manner, it creates challenges for permanency and the child's well-being. Until recently, no specific guidelines around SIJS existed in New Mexico. Individual caseworkers were responsible for identifying and applying for SIJS for eligible children, and it is suspected that over time some eligible children emancipated or were adopted from the foster care system without obtaining legal permanency resident status, leaving them with an undocumented status.

Immigration Liaison

PSD has responded aggressively to the need for a specialized set of skills and a deeper understanding of legal requirements concerning the immigrant population with the creation of a centralized immigration liaison position. In the past year, the immigration liaison has provided training statewide to all workers on best practice in working with immigrant families and forms of immigration relief available. The liaison has served as a coach and resource to front-line workers in staffing cases in terms of immigration and cultural issues, has assisted in locating interpretation services, and translated key documents. The liaison has provided consultation in evaluating eligibility and pursuing immigration relief for children and families involved in the system. The liaison has served as a referral source for immigration assistance and a link to governmental agencies such as foreign consulates, United States Citizenship and Immigration Services (USCIS), and ICE.

In considering the most successful practices around the country and needs in New Mexico, PSD designated the immigration liaison to manage all SIJS applications involving undocumented children in custody. The immigration liaison plays a key role in the SIJS process, and communicates with the caseworker and child, if appropriate, throughout the entire process. If any risk to applying is identified, the immigration liaison consults with an immigration attorney as to how to proceed with the application. The immigration liaison files the application as the child's representative. The liaison also attends USCIS adjustment of status interview as the child's representative with the child and the caseworker.

The role of the immigration liaison continues to expand as efforts are made to engage community partners in providing resources and assistance in cases involving immigrant families. PSD has recently partnered with a state university to create the capacity for law students specializing in immigration law to participate in student internships to assist with SIJS cases under the supervision of PSD's legal department and immigration liaison. The agency has also initiated communications with local USCIS offices in New Mexico to provide training to PSD staff on the process and required documentation for obtaining various forms of immigration relief available to immigrant clients.

Central Data Tracking System

PSD has developed a centralized tracking system to collect data on key case variables to identify patterns and ongoing needs in working with immigrants in various demographic areas of the state. The purpose of this database is to collect information concerning immigrant children and families in order to assist in determining eligibility for certain benefits and programs, comply with requirements for consular notification, and best utilize all available specialized resources to serve them. Data on undocumented children in custody is obtained through an existing internal data report on Title IV-E eligibility by filtering for a code designated for IV-E ineligible children due to legal status. Data on other non-U.S. citizen children and parents is compiled from various reporting sources. Copies of all consular notification forms regarding legal status for parents and children are provided by field offices to the immigration liaison. PSD's Title IV-E specialists send reports on parent and child legal status to the immigration liaison when determining IV-E eligibility at the onset of a case. In addition, local county office management sends monthly reports to the immigration liaison updating to their lists of cases involving foreign nationals. The immigration liaison utilizes all of these reporting sources to compile and verify the legal status of parents and their children in care.

CONCLUSION

Although PSD has made tremendous progress in establishing formal mechanisms to address the increasing needs of immigrant families in the child welfare system, the work is far from complete. One long-term goal is to integrate data regarding immigration into the central statewide data management system for federal reporting in order to ensure greater reliability of the data collected.

Another work in progress lies in addressing barriers to effective service on the border. It is imperative that PSD receive collaboration from divisions of DHS and establish mutual protocols on specific border issues impacting the child welfare system. These protocols might include permission for border crossing cards for court hearings, medical appointments, and visits; visits at the CBP Port of Entry buildings; immunity to state child welfare workers for transport of undocumented children in custody of the state; procedures for an official exchange of children at border crossing between New Mexico and Mexico child welfare agencies; and collaboration in scheduled immigration raids so that PSD is prepared to respond.

PSD is also exploring the possibility of establishing official protocols with DIF, the national child welfare agency in Mexico, and hospitals in New Mexico regarding "border babies," to reinforce the position that abuse cases involving babies born in U.S. hospitals on the border to Mexican nationals who do not reside in the United States be directed to DIF, unless DIF identifies that the baby would not be safe if returned to family members or kin in Mexico. Such a protocol would also need to address cases of Mexican children whose families reside in Mexico who are receiving medical care at U.S. hospitals. Ideally, this protocol would also include a stipulation that directs schools in U.S. border towns to contact DIF directly for concerns about the home lives of children living in Mexico who attend school in the United States.

PSD continues to explore opportunities to offer advanced and ongoing training within the agency on issues regarding immigrant children and families, effective practices, and federal and state laws that affect them. PSD also recognizes the need to augment targeted training for bilingual and bicultural staff to create expert workers and streamline cases involving immigrants in every region of the state to increase the ability to provide quality services.

While multidisciplinary immigrant outreach events are becoming more common across the state, it would be beneficial to expand PSD's use of positions that involve community outreach to develop more connections with immigrant community service providers. PSD would also benefit from increasing targeted efforts to involve immigrant community members in citizen review boards, Court Appointed Special Advocates, and recruitment of foster and adoptive parents in the immigrant community.

The New Mexico child welfare system struggles with ongoing challenges in the intersection of child welfare and migration that are well documented across the nation, and also possesses a unique border state perspective. New Mexico has made significant strides in recent years in adapting the child welfare system to enhance response and intervention with immigrant families in the state through changes to policy, procedure and organization, and through strengthening cross-disciplinary partnerships with immigrant serving agencies. Though the work is not complete, PSD has a plan of action to diligently address the barriers that remain, has identified a clear set of goals to be achieved, and will continue to engage public and private partners to reinforce the strengthening of and advocacy for immigrant families in New Mexico.

NOTES

1. For specific examples of media coverage of immigration enforcement activities in New Mexico, please contact the author.
2. In one case, PSD received custody of a US citizen child directly from ICE on the detainment and eventual deportation of the child's mother in their home. This mother had not committed serious crimes, but the PSD worker was informed by the ICE agent that the agent was required to give custody of US-citizen children to the local child welfare agency on detainment of an undocumented parent.
3. To obtain examples of policy examples or copies of public documents, please contact the author.

REFERENCES

Alderete, E., Vega, W., Kolody, B., & Aguilar-Gaxiola, S. (1999). Depressive symptomology: Prevalence and psychosocial risk factors among Mexican migrant farmworkers in California. *Journal of Community Psychology, 27,* 457–471.

Annie E. Casey Foundation (2009). *KIDS COUNT Data center: New Mexico percentage of children in immigrant families.* Retrieved from http://datacenter.kidscount. org/data/bystate/Rankings.aspx?state=NM&ind=3799

Basch, L., Glick-Schiller, N., & Szanton-Blanc, C. (1994). *Nations abound: Transnational projects, postcolonial predicaments, and deterritorialized nation-states.* Amsterdam, The Netherlands: Gordon and Breach Science Publishers.

Borelli, K., Earner, I., & Lincroft, Y. (2008). Administrators in public child welfare: Responding to immigrant families in crisis. *Protecting Children, 22*(2), 8–19.

Capps, R., Castaneda, R. M., Chaudry, A., & Santos, R. (2007). *Paying the price: The impact of immigration raids on America's children.* Washington, DC: The Urban Institute.

Capps, R., Fix, M., Ost, J., Reardon–Anderson, J., & Passel, J. (2004). *The health and well–being of young children of immigrants.* Washington, DC: Urban Institute.

Capps, R., & Fortuny, K. (2006). *Immigration and child and family policy.* Washington, DC: Urban Institute.

Capps, R., & Passel, J. (2004). *Describing immigrant communities.* New York, NY: Foundation for Child Development.

Chaudry, A., Capps, R., Pedroza, J. M., Castaneda, R. M., Santos, R., & Scott, M. (2009). *Facing our future: Children in the aftermath of immigration enforcement.* Washington, DC: The Urban Institute.

Coltrane, S., Parke, R., & Adams, M. (2004). Complexity of father involvement in low–income Mexican American families. *Family Relations, 53,* 179–189.

Cunradi, C., Caetano, R., and Shafer, J. (2002). Socioeconomic predictors of intimate partner violence among white, black, and Hispanic couples in the United States. *Journal of Family Violence, 17,* 377–389.

Dettlaff, A. & Rycraft, J. (2006). The impact of migration and acculturation on Latino children and families: Implications for child welfare practice. *Protecting Children, 21*(2), 6–21.

Dettlaff, A., Vidal de Haymes, M., Velazquez, S., Mindell, R., & Bruce, L. (2009). Emerging issues at the intersection of immigration and child welfare: Results from a transnational research and policy forum. *Child Welfare, 88*(2), 47–67.

Earner, I. (2005). Immigrant children and youth in the child welfare system—Immigration status and special needs in permanency planning. In G. Mallon & P. Hess (Eds.), *Child welfare in the 21st century: A handbook of practices, policies and programs.* New York, NY: Columbia University Press.

Earner, I. (2007). Immigrant families and child welfare: Barriers to services and approaches to change. *Child Welfare, 88*(3), 63–91.

Finch, B., Frank, R., and Vega, W. (2004). Acculturation and acculturation stress: A social-epidemiological approach to Mexican migrant farmworkers' health. *International Migration Review, 38,* 236–262.

Finno, M., Reyes, G., Espinoza Rodriguez, G., & Gallardo Robles, E. (2010, January). *Mexican minors in protective services: Intergovernmental partnerships and innovative practices*. Paper presented at 2010 New Mexico Children's Law Institute, Albuquerque, NM.

Fontes, L. (2002). Child discipline and physical abuse in immigrant Latino families: Reducing violence and misunderstandings. *Journal of Counseling and Development, 80*, 31–40.

Fong, R. (Ed.). (2004). *Culturally competent practice with immigrant and refugee children and families*. New York, NY: Guilford Press.

Georgia Department of Human Resources Division of Family and Children Services. (2009). *Working with immigrant children and families: A practice model*. Retrieved from http://www.hunter.cuny.edu/socwork/nrcfcpp/info_services/immigration–and–child–welfare.html

Hancock, T. (2005). Cultural competence in the assessment of poor Mexican families in the rural southeastern United States. *Child Welfare, (84)*, 689–711.

Hovey, J. (2000). Acculturative stress, depression, and suicidal ideation in Mexican immigrants. *Cultural Diversity and Ethnic Minority Psychology, 6*(2), 134–151.

Leon, A., & Dziegielewski, S. (1999). The psychological impact of migration: Practice considerations in working with Hispanic women. *Journal of Social Work Practice, 13*(1), 69–82.

Lincroft, Y., Resner, J., Leung, M., & Bussiere, A. (2006). *Undercounted, underserved: Immigrant and refugee families in the child welfare system*. Baltimore, MD: Annie E. Casey Foundation

Miranda, A., & Matheny, K. (2000). Sociopsychological predictors of acculturative stress among Latino adults. *Journal of Mental Health Counseling, 22*(4), 306–317.

New Mexico Children's Code: NMSA, §§ 32A–1–1 *et. seq* (1978).

New Mexico Children, Youth and Families Department. (2009). *PSD's Mission, Vision and Principles*. Retrieved from http://www.cyfd.org

New Mexico Legislature (2009). *HB0428: Prohibition of Profiling Practices Act*. Retrieved from http://www.nmlegis.gov/Sessions/09%20Regular/final/HB0428.pdf

New Mexico Voices for Children. (2007). *Immigration in New Mexico: A KIDS COUNT special report*. Albuquerque, NM: Author.

New York City Administration for Children's Services. (2005). *Immigration and language guidelines for child welfare staff* (2nd ed.). Retrieved from http://www.nyc.gov

Olayo Mendez, J. (2006). Latino parenting expectations and style: A literature review. *Protecting Children, 21*(2), 53–61.

Padilla, A., & Perez, W. (2003). Acculturation, social identity, and social cognition: A new perspective. *Hispanic Journal of Behavioral Sciences, 25*(1), 35–55.

Partida, J. (1996). The effects of immigration on children in the Mexican American community. *Child and Adolescent Social Work Journal, 13*(3), 241–254.

Passel, J. (2005). *Estimates of the size and characteristics of the undocumented population*. Washington, DC: Pew Hispanic Center.

Passel, J. (2006). *The size and characteristics of the unauthorized population in the U.S.* Washington, DC: Pew Hispanic Center.

Passel, J., & Cohn, D. (2009). *A portrait of unauthorized immigrants in the United States*. Washington, DC: Pew Hispanic Center.

Pine, B. A., & Drachman, D. (2005). Effective child welfare practice with immigrant and refugee children and their families. *Child Welfare, 84*, 537–562.

Solis, J. (2003). Re–thinking illegality as a violence against, not by Mexican immigrants, children, and youth. *Journal of Social Sciences, 59*, 15–31.

Smart, J., & Smart, D. (1995). Acculturative stress of Hispanics: Loss and challenge. *Journal of Counseling and Development, 73*, 390–396.

State of New Mexico (2008, May). *Impact of immigration raids on children and the state child welfare response.* Presented at U.S. House of Representatives Committee on Education and Labor, Subcommittee on Workforce Protections, Washington, DC.

State of New Mexico (2009a). *SIJS instructional and training guide* [unpublished training document]. Santa Fe, NM: Author.

State of New Mexico (2009b). *Working with immigrants in protective services: PSD protective services mandatory annual training 2009* [unpublished training document]. Santa Fe, NM: Author.

Thoman, L., & Suris, A. (2004). Acculturation and acculturative stress as predictors of psychological distress and quality–of–life functioning in Hispanic psychiatric patients. *Hispanic Journal of Behavioral Sciences, 26*(3), 293–311.

University of New Mexico Corinne Wolfe Children's Law Center (2007). *Child protection best practices bulletin: Working with undocumented and mixed status immigrant children and families.* Albuquerque, NM: Author.

United States Census Bureau. (2006). *2006 American Community Survey.* Retrieved from http://factfinder.census.gov

Velasquez, S., Vidal de Haymes, M., & Mindell, R. (2006). Migration: A critical issue for child welfare. *Protecting Children, 21*(2), 2–4.

Vericker, T., Kuehn, D., & Capps, R. (2008). Latino children of immigrants in the Texas child welfare system. *Protecting Children, 22*(2), 1–21.

Vidal de Haymes, M. (2005). Addressing the child welfare needs of immigrant and mixed–status families: Collaborative partnerships in Illinois that bridge organizational, community, and national borders to serve Latino families. *Protecting Children, 20*(1), 16–27.

Zielewski, E., Malm, K., & Geen, R. (2006). *Children caring for themselves and child neglect: When do they overlap?* Washington DC: Urban.

Using Simulation Training to Improve Culturally Responsive Child Welfare Practice

ROBIN LEAKE, KATHLEEN HOLT
CATHRYN POTTER and DEBORA M. ORTEGA

Child welfare professionals need to understand the complexities of the factors that influence parenting, values, and worldviews. Being able to work across cultures is critical to assessing safety, obtaining effective services, and creating permanent healthy families for children of color. The purpose of the project was to grapple with the challenge of increasing culturally responsive practice in a context of safety and permanency that is defined by American political and cultural values. The response to this challenge was a competency-based training program designed to enhance the effectiveness of child welfare practice with Latino families. A key feature of the training was a simulation to raise awareness and learning readiness through an experiential approach to learning. The simulation is the first component of a multi-faceted training curriculum aimed at the integration of culturally responsive practices in child welfare practice. The training series was part of a 3-year demonstration project funded by the Children's Bureau (Washington, DC).

Latino[1] families are the fastest growing and youngest population in the United States. Approximately 40% of the Latino population is younger than age 19 years (Pew Hispanic Center, 2006). Consequently, Latinos make up a growing number of families in American society and in the American child welfare systems (Child Welfare League of America, 2003). Like other minority groups, Latinos experience disproportionate socioeconomic risks and child welfare outcomes, including facing helping professionals with little knowledge of their culture and social experiences. Latinos also experience unique challenges associated with the changing landscape of opinions and policies related to immigration. At the same time, engaging child welfare workers in cultural responsiveness training can trigger resistance that interferes with skill development. This article describes a creative approach to preparing child welfare workers for cultural responsiveness training using a large-scale simulation of a community. In addition, the results of the formative evaluation, recommendations for further evaluation and implications for practice are presented.

BACKGROUND

Research indicates that minority families experience disproportionate environmental risk factors. The data collected for Latinos through the census and other sources is historically inaccurate (Ortega, 2009). Most scholars believe that information underrepresents the actual number of Latinos experiencing poverty and involved in the child welfare system (Salazar, Bornstein-Gomez, Mercado, Martinez, Ortega, Somoza, et al., 2008; Zambrana & Dorrington, 1998). While the Adoption and Foster Care Analysis Reporting System (AFCARS) collects data on Latinos as a distinct group, confusion about race and ethnicity variables lead to inaccurate reporting (Suleiman, 2003). Nonetheless, Latinos are three times more likely to be poor than their white counterparts (Perez, 2004).

These vulnerable families not only experience high levels of poverty, but also have limited resources (i.e., education, access to health care, underemployment, immigration status) (Zambrana & Dorrington, 1998). This combination of factors results in a number of obstacles that influence access to social service organizations (National Council of La Raza, 2008; Salazar et al., 2008; Suleiman, 2003; Zambrana & Dorrington, 1998). For Latinos who have limited English proficiency, the lack of bilingual service providers, limited access to interpreters, and lack of training for providers in the use of interpreters may jeopardize the safety of children and family reunification (Suleiman, 2003).

Rates of Latino children involved with the child welfare system have doubled since 1990, and Latinos are already overrepresented in the child welfare system in many states (United States Department of Health and

Human Services, 2003). The Adoption and Safe Families Act of 1997 (ASFA) legislates the provision of service that guards the safety, permanency, and well being of families, and requires accountability for these values from the states. The cultural barriers facing Latino families may threaten our ability to assure that the values of ASFA are being enacted. For example, safety is difficult to assure if the worker has limited understanding of the cultural context in which she is assessing safety. Language difficulties, cross-cultural misunderstandings, and fear of involvement with authorities make it difficult to identify kinship and other informal resources that contribute to timely permanency. Conducting a social history without both historical and current context presents challenges to professionals working from a competency-based framework (Santiago-Rivera, Arredondo, & Gallardo-Cooper, 2002).

Understanding the effects of political, economic, and unique cultural aspects of family functioning is critical to assessing safety and providing effective services that ensure permanence and well-being for Latino families. Numerous training and program initiatives have provided the knowledge and exposure to practices that are family centered, yet many workers are left frustrated by system barriers and lack of experience in successfully implementing skills across cultures.

CULTURAL RESPONSIVENESS TRAINING

The need for service providers to have increased cultural sensitivity, specific knowledge of the cultural/ethic groups they serve, and culturally responsive helping skills has been firmly established (Leong & Wagner, 1994). However, the best training methods for teaching these competencies are still largely unknown (Cashwell, 1994). Most cultural responsiveness training available to child welfare professionals focuses on acquiring knowledge about particular cultural groups. This, coupled with the desire of workers to have a "recipe card" approach to understanding complex cultural features, can foster false assumptions or stereotypes related to language, religious affiliation, immigration status, and citizenship (Santiago-Rivera et al., 2002). In addition, while much training focuses on knowledge and understanding about cultural differences, little is available that supports ongoing self-reflection and dialogue as precursors to teaching skills for working with diverse families.

Numerous studies about human services training indicate that participants rarely apply the knowledge and skills learned in a training setting to the job environment (Baer Wells, Rosengren, Hartzler, Beadnell, et al., 2009; Curry, Caplan, & Knuppel, 1994; Wehrmann, Shin, & Poertner, 2002). Referred to as the "transfer problem," some researchers estimate that only 10%–20% of what is taught in training actually transfers to the job (Baldwin & Ford, 1988). Studies over the past 20 years have shown that factors associated with personal attributes, training design, and work environment predict how training participants transfer knowledge and skills to the job. Individual attributes that predict transfer include motivation, learning readiness, and perceived utility (Baldwin & Ford, 1988; Curry et al., 1994). Conversely, training participants who lack personal interest in the training are less likely to transfer the knowledge and skills to the job (Miller & Rollnick, 2002).

Training programs designed to increase multicultural awareness and culturally responsive practice are especially resistant to transfer (Brown, 2004). Studies of multicultural pre-service training for teachers found that training failed to change stereotyped perceptions of themselves and others (Banks, 2001). One reason might be that people are naturally resistant to confronting long-held beliefs about self and others (Allport, 1979). This resistance is operationalized in the classroom setting by lack of preparation, engagement and commitment, and participation in activities (Irvine, 1992). Thus, instructional methods that reduce natural resistance to modifying strongly held belief systems are important for transfer of learning. Educational experts believe that effective multicultural training must engage participants in examining their own self-concepts, history, and current belief systems and in developing an understanding and respect for other cultures (Brown, 1998).

Cultural training often focuses on providing knowledge about culture, ethnicity, racism, and disproportionality. While instructional strategies that teach facts and promote knowledge about minority cultures are valuable, many studies have demonstrated the importance of experiential learning in helping students connect the curriculum content and message in a meaningful way (Brown, 2004).

The desire for human service workers to have a step-by-step process for working with diverse families has been fueled by educational and training approaches that are based on essentialist models of teaching about cultural groups. Essentialist approaches, in addition to reducing culture to finite characteristics (i.e., all Latinos are late because they have a different time orientation) reinforce the perspective that people who are influenced by more than United States culture are so different that they are "alien." The exotification of cultural differences can create a barrier to empathy if workers' understanding of diverse people is limited to concretized boxes of generalized cultural characteristics. This limiting approach to understanding culture, coupled with the often-held fear by workers that they may display racist thinking or behaviors, can create more barriers that interfere with the helping process.

Empathy provides helping professionals with a deeper understanding of the experiences and challenges of the people they serve. Empathy becomes the vehicle through which the child welfare professional can relate to barriers, misperceptions, and misunderstanding about people whose cultures may be different from their own. To the extent that practitioners attending training about culture are more empathetic to the challenges faced by ethnic minority clients, motivation to learn skills to serve these families may increase. In turn, participants who are motivated, ready to learn, and see the connection between the training and their job are more likely to apply the clinical skills they learn in training to their job (Antle, Barbee, & van Zyl, 2008).

One way to teach empathy is through designed scenarios that allow participants to experience the life of another through experiential simulation. According to one researcher, "empathy is a vitally important aspect of both experiential learning and good therapy" (Browning, Collins, & Nelson, 2005, p. 4). In a role-play activity, the training participant takes the role of a hypothetical person with a specific personality, history or context (Browning et al., 2005). One study found that medical students who were taught empathy using an experiential simulation were more likely to retain skills over time compared with students who were taught empathy through a discussion group (Rae & Willis, 1973). Role-play is also a method for culture-specific training because experiential exercises improve multicultural skills, awareness, and knowledge (Brown, 2004; Helmeke & Prouty, 2001; Minor, 1983).

Role-play provides the service provider with a platform for considering and discussing cultural issues and encourages a deeper level of empathetic understanding of the experiences of others (Brathwaite & Majumdar, 2006; Cashwell, Looby, & Housley, 1997; Harter, 1981; Helmeke & Prouty, 2001; Kim & Lyons, 2003). One study found that pre-service teachers who engaged in experiential simulations were better able to put themselves "in the shoes of others" and experience the effects of minority status (Brown, 2004). Participating in role-play exercises with people from different cultural backgrounds also increases therapists' sensitivity and comfort with working with diverse clients (Helmeke & Prouty, 2001). While role-play as an experiential learning strategy has been clearly demonstrated and widely used in the field of multicultural counseling (Kim & Lyons, 2003; Torres Jr. & Ottens, 1997), there are few experiential-based training programs that address cultural responsiveness in child welfare.

The term *experiential simulation* describes more complex role-play situations with multiple characters, scripted situations and socioemotional family histories, and often involves props. Simulations allow training participants to experience a character with more depth and nuance than traditional role-play, thus increasing empathy (Shepard, 2002). The use of multiple characters allows participants to interact and experience more dynamic and complex social situations (Browning et al., 2005). When participants have adequate time to prepare themselves for their roles, they are more likely to stay in character by relying on feelings of empathy and the social history provided for their character. Experiential simulations can lead to powerful emotions that translate into greater empathy and understanding for people who differ from themselves (Browning et al., 2005).

THE PROGRAM MODEL

The Child Welfare Resource Network, at the School of Social Welfare of the University of Kansas, developed a comprehensive, research–driven competency-based training program titled *Effective Child Welfare Practice with Latino Families*. The series incorporates several best practices in training: 1) Agency and community investment in training development; 2) focus on skill development based on experiential learning through self-reflection and dialog; and 3) extension of training events over time to facilitate practice, review and debriefing (see Figure 2). The training modules are supported by pre- and post-training elements, culturally relevant materials, and a comprehensive resource guide. A National Advisory Committee with expertise in multiculturalism, Latino immigration issues and culturally responsive child welfare practice developed the framework for the training and curriculum content.

A critical piece of the curriculum series and the focus of this article is *El Jardin* (The Garden), a half-day simulation designed to provide workers with the opportunity to understand the experience of Latino client families in the child welfare system. The simulation addresses some of the poor practice behaviors that develop out of the lack of fit between social systems and Latino client families and desirable practice responses and behaviors. *El Jardin* fosters the development of an empathetic understanding of the range of Latino experiences, motivates workers to develop their knowledge and skills to work with Latino families, and expose areas of unintended system or personal bias. The simulation closes with action planning informed by self-reflection, engagement, and dialogue to support the cultural responsiveness that serves as a "springboard" for the remainder of the skills-based training.

The *El Jardin* simulation was based on methodology developed by Wentz and Gerber (2009) who have used simulation with independent living for youth, collaborative case staffing, and courtroom performance. Figure 1 illustrates a process that begins with elaboration of the central theme or area of focus. Goals are developed to define cognitive, affective, and psychomotor outcomes for participants. Sub-themes are woven throughout the scripts, the characters, and the time frames that comprise the simulation. Characters in the simulation vary by age, gender, and life experiences. Scenarios for each character are designed to allow participants to experience a full range of emotion, including hope, frustration, motivation, and social pressures as they engage in best and less-than-best practice behavior (R. Wentz & N. Gerber, personal communication, May 2008).

Once the simulation goals have been established, developers build the environment, establish roles, family scenarios, activities, challenges, and scripted behavioral responses. The simulation scenarios were collaboratively developed by the trainers, advisory group members and practitioners in Kansas and Colorado and informed by best practice literature. Efforts were

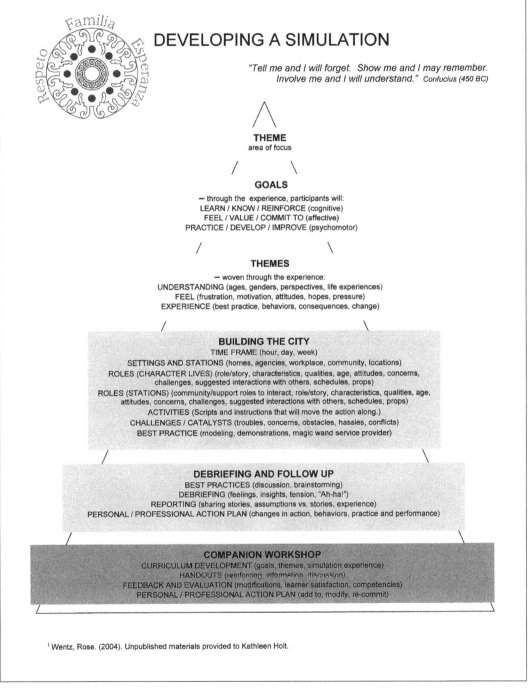

FIGURE 1 Developing a Simulation.

Part I—El Jardin: A Simulation Highlighting Latino Families' Experience with Community Based Services & Foundations for Culturally Responsive Practice with Latino Families is a two segment, one-day training. The morning simulation is an experiential learning activity designed to help participants develop a insight and understanding into the lives and service needs of Latino families. The afternoon workshop session includes discussion of cultural responsiveness, the need for on-going self-reflection/assessment, the strengths of Latino culture, and the barriers to service faced by many Latino families.

Part II—Core Elements of Culturally Responsive Practice with Latino Families is a two day training series designed to explore the elements and skills to promote safety and permanency in Latino Families. Participants will explore demographics, traditions of Latino culture, citizenship and immigration, working with translators, developing the skills of cross-cultural service provision and defining best practice working with Latino families.

Part III—Developing a Culturally Responsive Team is a one-day workshop for agency supervisors to encourage an agency culture that promotes skill development in culturally responsive practice. The afternoon features presentation of three videos designed to be used with in-service or brown bag discussions.

Part IV—Advanced Topics include three video productions for in-service, classroom or "brown bag" presentations to be facilitated by local/regional "experts." The topics include From the Field—Immigration & Child Welfare; Domestice Violence Dynamics in Immigrant Communities; and Legal Options for Immigrant & Foreign-born Victims.

Part V—Teaching Effective Practice with Hispanic Families: Curriculum modules for Social Work Departments includes awareness and skill building exercises for social work faculty. The exercises are designed to supplement existing course offerings.

FIGURE 2 Effective Child Welfare Practice with Latino Families Training Series.

made to ensure that the simulation was aligned with community demographics to ensure an authentic experience for training participants. Simulations are set up using conference style tables and chairs with community stations around the room and families in the center of the room. For *El Jardin*, up to 55 participants were grouped into five families, community members and providers. *El Jardin* includes experiences of third-generation families, immigrant families with documentation, mixed immigration status families, speakers of indigenous languages, and non-Latino neighbors and providers (Figure 3). Extensive props provide emotional relief and distance as well as encourage participants to remain in character while experiencing stressful circumstances such as teen pregnancy, detention, safety assessments, and court appearances. The challenges, troubles, concerns, obstacles, and conflicts serve as catalysts for action, understanding, and empathy (R. Wentz & N. Gerber, personal communication, May 2008).

Violeta Family (County of origin: Mexico)

Family members: Victor (dad); Valeria (mom); Valencia (4 years); Vanessa (18 months); Victoria (newborn).

Scenario/Issues: Parents undocumented immigrants with one-foreign- and two United States-born daughters. Father believes children born in the United States will prevent deportation. Underemployed and frustrated with low pay, he begins to carry drugs to make more money. Fight with wife ensues. A domestic violence call results in law enforcement discovering presence of controlled substances. Parents are detained at Immigration and Customs Enforcement (ICE) and the children are placed in foster care. Dad faces deportation. Mom may be eligible to remain under Violence Against Women Act (VAWA) if she cooperates with authorities as a witness against dad. Issues include immigration laws/practices, domestic violence, placement, and legal rights.

Amarillo Family (County of origin: El Salvador)

Family members: Arturo (dad); Arcadia (mom); Alberto (16 years, nephew); Azura (12 years); Alejandro (10 years).

Scenario/Issues: Recently their 16-year-old nephew moved to *El Jardin* to live with the family in a kinship arrangement due to gang activity. The two birth children are acculturating, but because their mother speaks little English, she is very worried about the influence of the neighborhood boys on her son in particular. Her harsh discipline involves keeping both children at home without food. Azura who admires the older girls in the neighborhood, has recently had a tattoo. Issues involve kinship, acculturation, generational differences in acculturation, language barriers, gang activity and youth behaviors, interacting with the school system, and discipline practices.

Naranja Family (Country of origin: Guatemala)

Family members: Nuncio (dad, in Guatemala); Norma (mom); Nicky (4 years); Navea (3 years).

Scenario/Issues: The father was recruited to come to the United States as a foreman on a work visa due to the fact that he speaks Kanjobal, a Guatemalan dialect and Spanish. He was able to bring his family over, but had to leave a newborn with his mother in Guatemala until he could obtain permission for both to join the family. He has returned to Guatemala where he is awaiting his mother's papers so the family can be reunited in the United States. His wife is extremely isolated since no one she knows in the United States speaks Kanjobal. She tries to find a *curandera*, but cannot and becomes so depressed that she fails to adequately supervise her children. Issues involve language barriers, health practices, isolation, supervision/discipline practices, and definitions of family. *(continued)*

FIGURE 3 The Families of *El Jardin*.

After the simulation, participants debrief in character using a diary format. Additionally, each participates in a group discussion in which they are asked to identify key learning points from the simulation. The afternoon session employs a more traditional workshop format to support open dialogue

Rojo Family (Country of origin: Mexico)

Family members: Roberto (dad); Raquel (mom); Rico (19 years); Rolanda (16 years, teen mom); Reyna (newborn baby of Rolanda); Ramon (11 years); Rosa (6 years); Reuben (2 years).

Scenario/Issues: Dad drinks heavily. Teen daughter has acculturation issues (parents want Rolanda to be responsible for all kids in home; she wants to be out with her American friends). Rolanda is a new teen mother. There have been physical altercations between Dad and Rolanda. Mom takes children out of school to translate for appointments. The family has been in the United States for years. Dad is a naturalized United States citizen; Mom is a permanent resident; children are United States citizens by derivation, except oldest son Rico (Mexican citizen) who just joined the family in the United States after living with his grandparents in Mexico. Issues involve the use of alcohol, generational acculturation, family roles, teen pregnancy, employment, citizenship and status, and father/daughter relationships.

MacGreene Family (Country of Origin: United States)

Family members: Melvin (foster dad); Maureen (foster mom); Mallory (15 years, daughter); Marta Mendoza (teen in foster care); Manuel and Marciel Martinez (godparents to Marta).

Scenario/Issues: Marta Mendoza and her boyfriend ran away from her mother's and stepfather's home in California. He abandoned her in *El Jardin*. She was placed in a newly licensed foster home where she refused to speak English. Foster mother believes Marta has an eating disorder, so takes her to the clinic where it is revealed that Marta is pregnant. Marta's godparents live in El Jardin and are second-generation citizens who direct programs through the local community center linked to the Catholic Church. Issues involve foster family preparation, language barriers, marital stress, god-parenting, teen pregnancy, and kinship definitions.

FIGURE 3 (*Continued*).

about insights and understanding gathered from the morning and to set the scene for ongoing self-reflection and action planning.

Training strategies were designed to promote active engagement and preparation and mitigate reluctance on the part of workers to engage in role play simulation. Pre-training materials include a brief description of *El Jardin*, including goals and objectives, and guidelines for participation. Participants are given a welcome packet at registration that includes a self-reflection survey, the tools for dialogue, and material describing the simulation. To emphasize the importance of participation and openness to learning, each participant is asked to sign a certificate of readiness indicating that he/she had read all materials and agrees to enter *El Jardin* ready to learn.

The companion workshop that completes *Foundations for Effective Practice with Latino Families* incorporates the goals and themes of the simulation into more content-oriented curriculum, using handouts and exercises building on the simulation tools for dialogue and self-reflection. Action plans and goals completed throughout the training series are supported through a series of follow-up electronic newsletters featuring short informational segments. Participants are reminded to continue practicing skills to promote transfer of learning. The *El Jardin* simulation was delivered four times in Kansas and three times in Colorado throughout the 3-year demonstration project.

Development costs for simulations may be higher than traditional training modules to the extent that they rely on a community-embedded process and elaborate props that support the experience. The replication of the simulation in a new setting requires the support of a team of local child welfare and community experts who can take the existing simulation framework and customize to local issues and environments. The materials budget for *El Jardin* was $3,400 (props, scripts, culturally relevant items such as worry dolls, *dichos*, or *milagros*), with implementation costs being similar to standard training deliveries, with the exception of the need for a larger space and two to four trainers who can play central roles and manage the experience.

EVALUATION APPROACH AND METHODS

The primary purpose of the evaluation was to provide meaningful formative feedback to the project team to guide the development of the training. Because this was a training demonstration project, most of the resources and time were directed toward developing and refining the training intervention. Because the training evolved over time, there was not a consistent product to assess until the very end of the project. Thus, the scope of the project did not include a study of training outcomes to evaluate learning and changes in attitude, knowledge, skills, and job behaviors. Nonetheless, the evaluation was able to describe how participants experienced the training and elicit some examples of how they transferred their learning to the job and improved their work with Latino families.

The evaluators worked closely with the project team to develop a communication strategy that facilitated an interactive process of immediate feedback followed by curriculum revision and refinement. The focus on formative measures such as qualitative observations and interviews and participant self-reports was an appropriate evaluation approach for the stage of development of the project. However, future evaluation will need to focus on long-term outcomes such as participant learning, transfer of learning to the job, and performance impact, in order to establish the effectiveness of the training model.

Methods

The formative training evaluation methods for this demonstration project included participant self-report through questionnaires administered at two time-points, focus groups, and structured interviews with professional observers from the project advisory board and the project staff.

TRAINING SATISFACTION SURVEY

Project staff administered a training satisfaction instrument to measure participant impressions of the effectiveness and importance of training, the expertise of the trainer, and the level of supervisory support for transfer of learning. The instrument was revised several times throughout the grant period as the training developed. The lack of consistency in instruments made it difficult to compare quantitative data across trainings. The evaluators analyzed the survey data by aggregating responses by common questions. Responses from 114 participants were included in the analysis. Participants provided qualitative responses to questions regarding satisfaction and importance.

FOLLOW-UP QUESTIONNAIRE

A 25-item on-line questionnaire was developed by University of Denver evaluators and administered to participants who attended any of the training modules—simulation/foundations, core, and advanced topics at the end of the 3-year grant project. The questionnaire asked participants to rate their learning on key training competencies and the extent to which they use their learning on their job, using a five-point Likert-style format with responses ranging from *strongly disagree* to *strongly agree*.

An email with a link to the survey using Survey Monkey (www.survey monkey.com) was sent to 282 participants, and 78 were returned as address unidentified, indicating that the participant was no longer with the agency, or perhaps the address was incorrect on the attendance spreadsheets. From a pool of 203 participants, 51 completed the questionnaire, for a response rate of 25%. The rate of response was not unexpected, considering that approximately half of the participants attended training over one year prior to the questionnaire being administered. However, the low rate of responses did not allow for the generalization of findings to the entire sample of training participants.

FOCUS GROUPS

Two focus groups were conducted at the end of the grant project, one in Garden City, Kansas, with 15 participants, and one in Alamosa, Colorado, with eight participants. Both child welfare agency staff and community partners attended the focus groups. Participants were asked about their experience with the simulation, suggestions for improvement, and transfer of learning opportunities.

At the end of the project, 15 individual 1-hour interviews were conducted with the project team, National Advisory Committee members, Local Advisory Board members, child welfare supervisors, training coordinators, and staff.

EVALUATION RESULTS

Satisfaction Survey Results

Aggregated responses from the training satisfaction survey administered immediately after the training suggest that participants felt that knowledge, attitudes, and skills improved as a result of the training. Specifically, at least 90% of participants reported learning in all key competency areas targeted by the training (Table 1).

Approximately 85% of participants strongly agreed that the training was important to their job, that they were motivated to use what they learned in training, and that they could see how they would transfer the learning to their

TABLE 1 Training Satisfaction: Knowledge, Attitudes, and Skills Learned in Training

Competency/Learning Objectives Participants can:	Mean	n	SD
1. Explain the importance of designing services to meet the needs of a rapidly growing number of Latino children.	3.55	114	.49
2. List three or more general cultural characteristics that may impact services without stereotyping Latino individuals or families.	3.40	102	.63
3. List two or more essential considerations in engaging Latino clients.	3.54	105	.57
4. Demonstrate use of ethnographic interviewing to conduct culturally responsive assessment.	3.60	78	.51
5. Understand the different types of immigration categories and conduct a basic assessment of the service eligibility of Latino individuals.	3.41	91	.57
6. List two elements of a plan for assisting Limited English Proficient persons.	3.44	108	.53
7. Articulate basic federal requirements for meaningful access to services for eligible applicants regardless of language preference.	3.33	92	.59
8. Explain the requirements for providing service to Limited English Proficient individuals.	3.35	91	.65
9. Demonstrate self-reflection and action planning to improve cultural-responsiveness.	3.54	111	.53

Note. Four-point Likert scale: 4 = strongly agree; 3 = agree; 2 = disagree; and 1 = strongly disagree.

job. Further, 82% strongly agreed that the training would make them more effective in their practice. The trainers also received high satisfaction ratings, with 95% of participants strongly agreeing that they trusted the trainers, the trainers sought their opinions and feedback, and they felt involved in the training.

When asked to identify what aspects of the training they liked the best through open-ended responses, participants identified the simulation as their top choice, followed by information about Latino culture and access to immigration resources, topics covered in the afternoon following the simulation. Many participants described in detail how the simulation raised their awareness of the language barriers and challenges faced by immigrant families. One participant wrote,

> I've done this work for more than three decades but when I needed a translator in order to help a young, scared pregnant girl, I just threw confidentiality out the window. I ran right out onto the street and grabbed the first person I could find to translate… I cannot believe I'd do something like that, but I did!

Another said,

> Even though the translator in El Jardin was pretending to translate from one language to another, even though I could understand every word that was said and every word as she pretended to translate it, it was amazing to feel scared knowing that others were talking about the future of my family!

Yet another said, "I was frustrated when they tried to offer me mental health when all I wanted was to talk to the priest or find a faith healer but they couldn't understand my language so it was a big problem."

Several participants noted that they found the simulation engaging and that it evoked strong emotions, even though they approached the exercise with skepticism and a dislike of role-play exercises. As one person noted,

> I don't like role playing so I chose a man who was in jail because I thought I would not do much, but when I was the character in jail I felt isolated and disappointed when my family couldn't all visit me and my AA meeting didn't happen.

Another noted,

> When I saw all the props, I was worried. I hate role playing, and I thought I would have to look stupid. I took a child's part so I wouldn't have to talk, but I discovered that I really got into it. Everyone was ignoring me and just pushing me to the side, and I actually experienced what that felt like. The simulation is powerful. I'll remember those feelings for a long time.

Even after the simulation was over and participants were completing their evaluations, they continued to write about their experiences in very personal terms, suggesting that the exercise effectively helped participants empathize with the characters they were portraying. One woman wrote, "I was so worried about my babies, I thought I would never see them again when they put me into detention." One male participant reported, "I didn't like not knowing what happened to my kids when I went to detention. No one told me anything and it was very frustrating." Still another looked forward, "I commit to looking at my own biases when it comes to working with Hispanic families and other families also seeing things through their eyes and hearing about the struggles they have encountered." From a participant playing a child's role came the following, "These are the struggles the families I work with deal with all the time. No wonder it's hard for them to go to school and concentrate."

Finally, participants reported gaining *new knowledge* in the simulation, mostly in regard to immigration issues:

- I always thought immigrants could get federal aid. I didn't know they needed to have documentation to be eligible.
- I am really amazed at how complicated immigration issues are but after the information shared at least I know now what to look for to help the families I work with.
- I never thought about the problems immigrants have getting services especially if they are undocumented.
- I had no idea there were medical services for immigrant families in our community.
- I didn't realize that people in detention can ask for a lawyer, but don't always get one and the immigration laws are so confusing. It would be easy to make a mistake that could affect a child or a parent forever. I definitely want to know more.

Participants evidenced motivation for further learning and for action, indicating that the training may have impacted readiness for learning. The final quote in the last paragraph illustrates this. Other comments included,

- I will work with my agency to look at how immigration policies impact the families we work with and create a committee to help others understand that deportation is not helpful.
- I will learn Spanish so I can further communicate with the families I work with.
- I want to learn more about immigration so I can help my undocumented families better.
- I work with Spanish-speaking people all the time and I thought there isn't anything new I could learn from this training (before the simulation). Wow!

I learned so much about my people (Latino) and the Spanish-speaking clients I work with.

- I thought, 'Great, another cultural responsive training!' but this was great. I learned so much, I am glad I came.

Participants also noted that the simulation helped to break down *community barriers*:

- It was great to sit at a table with people from other agencies and from other cultures as well. I learned much about both.
- This is the first time all these people from all of these agencies have sat at the same table. There is a lot of tension in our communities. We need to continue this dialog.

One participant put these themes together in a poignant story of self-examination:

> I told my supervisor that I needed to come to this training because, quite frankly I have a BIG problem working with Latino people and I didn't know why. This was probably the BEST training I've ever attended. I just realized that I have been so angry about people not speaking English. As I sat there and listened and talked, I remembered the many stories of my brothers being beat[en] at Haskell Indian School. They were beat for speaking our Potawamie language and all these years, I have grieved the loss of my native language, but I'd NEVER have spoken about it because I didn't want to get beat[en] for it like my brothers did. I learned so much about myself today.

Follow-up Survey Results

Approximately 90% of the respondents to the follow-up questionnaire administered at the completion of the project agreed or strongly agreed that they gained knowledge, understanding, and skills in most of the competency areas, with mean scores ranging from 3.53 to 4.36 on a five-point Likert-type scale, with 1 being strongly disagree and 5 being strongly agree (Table 2).

Focus Group and Interview Results

Participants were overwhelmingly positive about the simulation, echoing many of the themes from individual respondents. According to one participant,

> The training as a whole was motivating in so many ways. As a person who works with families of all backgrounds, I feel like I can communicate more comfortably with them. I even learned a great amount about my own personal heritage.

TABLE 2 Follow-up Questionnaire: Knowledge, Attitudes, and Skills Gains after Training

Competency/Learning Objective Participants can:	Mean	n	SD
1. I have a better understanding of the challenges that Spanish-speaking families face living in a monolingual society.	4.14	49	.89
2. I have a better understanding of immigration laws and policies.	3.60	44	.96
3. I have a better understanding of Hispanic/Latino culture.	4.00	48	.90
4. I have a better understanding of how immigration laws have impacted families' experiences with the child welfare system.	3.79	57	.96
5. I consider cultural traits when making decisions about families (i.e., familia, collectivism, spirituality, machismo, etc.)	4.39	46	.71
6. Cultural traits and characteristics shape my approach when working with families.	4.32	47	.76
7. I ask more questions about a family's culture, history, and background when interviewing.	4.00	44	.98
8. I know where to go to find culturally responsive services in my community.	3.87	46	.88
9. I am able to advocate effectively for services for Latino families in my caseload.	4.00	51	.75
10. I do more self-reflection of how my personal experiences and values impact my practice.	4.11	46	.77
11. I connect more families to language services.	3.66	41	1.0
12. My supervisor supports my efforts to be culturally responsive to families.	4.36	45	.68
13. I have made the changes that I identified in my "action plan" on the self-assessment form.	3.93	44	.85
14. I have used the handouts and materials provided in the training for reference.	3.53	47	1.1

Note. Five-point Likert-type scale: 5 = strongly agree; 4 = agree; 3 = neutral; 2 = disagree; and 1 = strongly disagree.

Those focus group participants who attended both simulation/foundations and core training reported that both modules were valuable, but that they particularly liked the simulation because it gave people a chance to feel some portion of what it was like to be a Latino family trying to navigate the system. As one participant in Wichita said,

> The best part was the role-play; lots of people came from different organizations who are not in direct services, so it was great that they got to experience a deeper understanding of the challenges Latinos face and how complicated things can get when there's a language barrier.

One Colorado supervisor felt that training was invaluable for enabling her workers to understand the struggles that their clients experience on a daily basis. "Once they feel what it's like, there's an 'ah ha' moment, and then they are motivated to learn more about cultural issues."

Another key finding was that the training offered child welfare workers the opportunity to network with other community providers who serve the same Latino families. Because of the intense emotional experience of the simulation and the group processing, participants felt that they forged relationships with community partners that impact the way they serve families. In one focus group in Garden City, a Head Start provider reported how she was inspired by the training to organize a "Mommy and Me" support group for Latino mothers. She called on several child welfare workers that she met in the training who now refer clients to her group. Project team staff confirmed that they have seen this powerful transformation over and over again. For example, after one simulation in Colorado, a family advocacy worker set up a planning session with a child welfare worker about conducting joint visits to families. Another participant started a bilingual unit at her agency that she continues to supervise. Many participants reported that their overall cultural sensitivity had increased as a result of the training.

Overall Findings

The results suggest that simulation training may be a promising approach for raising participants' awareness and understanding of the experience of Latino families, and especially immigrant families, in the child welfare system. This increased awareness appeared to be the first stage of readiness to explore their own biases and motivation for learning. Findings demonstrate that participants appreciated the simulation experience for opening their eyes to the challenges faced by Latino families, and were motivated to learn more about serving Latino families and apply their skills to providing more effective case practice.

Limitations of the Evaluation and Recommendations for Future Studies

As previously discussed, it is impossible to draw conclusions about the effectiveness of the training in raising awareness and improving skills in culturally based practice from these results. The evaluation was designed to gather formative feedback about the design and delivery of the training, and create a continuous feedback loop so that the project team could make ongoing improvements. These results do suggest, however, that many participants experienced this training to be profoundly different than other trainings about cultural competency, and that it was successful in raising their awareness of cultural issues with the Latino families they serve. Further, those who responded to the online questionnaire (for some, this was more than 1 year after they attended the training) said they clearly remembered this training more than others they have attended, and that the simulation changed their case practice. In light of these findings, the authors recommend that next steps include evaluating outcomes of simulation training to determine how simulation affects awareness and readiness for skills training. Ideally, the research design would compare the simulation model (a training simulation combined with skills-based training) with traditional training (just the skills-based training component) to test whether simulation leads to increased readiness and how readiness predicts learning and transferring of skills to the job. Methods should include a pre-post self-assessment and knowledge test, and a follow-up performance measure of transfer of learning.

DISCUSSION

The nature of child welfare work can make it difficult for workers to develop skills in serving Latino families. Training on cultural responsiveness often focuses on listing the generalized cultural characteristics of a particular minority group. Instead of a focus on building skills for multi-culturally responsive practice, training too often adopts a "tell us about them" approach that focuses on short-cuts for working with clients that are culturally different (Santiago-Rivera et al., 2002). In the crisis-oriented environment of many child welfare agencies, few workers develop the skills that would best promote understanding, foster engagement, and lead to effective practice. Role models for effective practice are few, and inexperienced workers do not always have opportunities to learn from experienced, culturally responsive mentors.

This project was designed with the premise that training can be structured to support the development of the beliefs and attitudes that open the door to increased knowledge and skill for cultural responsiveness. Child welfare professionals need the opportunity to experience what it is like to be Latino in the communities they serve. They need to feel the dilemmas that new immigrant families, migrant families, and fifth-generation Latino families feel in American society. Child welfare professionals need to understand the importance of practicing the skills of self-reflection, engaging, assessing, planning, and intervening with Latino families. Finally, child welfare professionals need opportunities to implement their new skills on the job with support from supervisors and colleagues. The pedagogical technique of training simulation to increase awareness, readiness, and motivation as a foundation for skill building is a promising approach in the field of cultural responsiveness training in child welfare.

Building a simulation experience requires that training teams engage in a collaborative learning process with agency, family, and community partners to identify and simulate the types of clients and issues faced by Latino families in the local community. In this way, a simulation like *El Jardin* is "tweaked" to capture and respond to local concerns. This does take time, however the process serves other important purposes as well, as trainers build upon community relationships and identify the important themes and sub-themes for inclusion. The task is to create a virtual reality that is separate enough to engage participants in role-play but familiar enough to be owned by participants. Engaging community partners and families in such an endeavor presents an opportunity to "build together." This is time consuming, but ultimately a more creative process than traditional knowledge training development. It is, indeed, more "real" for training developers and for participants.

The customization and embedding of a simulation into the local environment is very likely to be critical for success. As *El Jardin* was developed, immigration enforcement was shifting from Immigration and Naturalization Service (INS) to Homeland Security's Immigration and Customs Enforcement (ICE), the largest investigatory arm of Homeland Security. In Colorado, ICE was actively pursuing large raids on meat packing plants, resulting in many families coming into contact with child welfare due to detention of parents. This theme was woven into *El Jardin* resulting in an important sense of immediacy. This immediacy of content and application may well contribute to the strong sense of reality within a simulation.

Simulation training can be resource intensive, relying on boxes of props, large training spaces, strong community partnerships, and trainer creativity and time. Findings from the formative evaluation indicate that stakeholders felt that the simulation was well worth the time and effort. More studies to compare simulation to traditional training techniques are needed to confirm whether the engagement, readiness, and learning outcomes are fully worth the investment.

NOTE

1. The terms *Latino* and *Hispanic* are not interchangeable or widely accepted. Each term reflects complex political issues about the origin of the label and the related meaning. For instance, the term *Hispanic* was imposed by the United States federal government for tracking of information and refers to Spanish speaking people. For a population of people whose identity is without an agreed-upon name, the larger question to consider is the consequences for empowerment and unity. *Latino* is predominately used here because it is the preference of one of the authors as the lesser of potentially oppressive labels.

REFERENCES

Allport, G. W. (1979). *The nature of prejudice* (25th ed.). Reading, MA: Addison–Wesley.

Antle, B. F., Barbee, A. P., & van Zyl, M. A. (2008). A comprehensive model for child welfare training evaluation. *Children and Youth Services Review, 30*, 1063–1080.

Baer, J. S., Wells, E. A., Rosengren, D. B., Hartzler, B., Beadnell, B., & Dunn, C. (2009). Agency context and tailored training in technology transfer: A pilot evaluation of motivational interviewing training for community counselors. *Journal of Substance Abuse Treatment, 37*(2), 191–202.

Baldwin, T. T., & Ford, J. K. (1988). Transfer of training: A review and directions for future research. *Personnel Psychology, 41,* 63–105.

Banks, J. A. (2001). *Cultural diversity and education: Foundations, curriculum, and teaching* (4th ed.). Boston, MA: Allyn & Bacon.

Brathwaite, A. C., & Majumdar, B. (2006). Evaluation of a cultural competence educational programme. *Journal of Advanced Nursing, 53,* 470–479.

Brown, E. L. (1998). *The relevance of self–concept and instructional design in transforming Caucasian preservice teachers' monocultured worldviews of multicultural perceptions and behaviors. Dissertation Abstracts International, 59*(7), A2450.

Brown, E. L. (2004). What precipitates change in cultural diversity awareness during a multicultural course. *Journal of Teacher Education, 55,* 325–340.

Browning, S., Collins, J. S., & Nelson, B. (2005). Creating families: A teaching technique for clinical training through role-playing. *Marriage & Family Review, 38*(4), 1–19.

Cashwell, C. (1994). Interpersonal process recall. In *Explicating the significant components of effective supervision,* L. D. Borders (ed.). Greensboro, NC: ERIC/CASS.

Cashwell, C., Looby, E. J., & Housley, W. (1997). Appreciating cultural diversity through clinical supervision. *Clinical Supervisor, 15,* 75–85.

Child Welfare League of America. (2003). *Children of color in the child welfare system: Overview, vision, and proposed action steps.* Retrieved from http://www.cwla.org/programs/culture/disproportionatestatement.pdf

Curry, D., Caplan, P., & Knuppel, J. (1994). Transfer of Training and Adult Learning (TOTAL). *Journal of Continuing Social Work Education, 6,* 8–14.

Harter, S. (1981). A new self–report scale of intrinsic versus extrinsic orientation in the classroom: Motivational and informational components. *Developmental Psychology, 17,* 300–312.

Helmeke, K. B., & Prouty, A. M. (2001). Do we really understand? An experiential exercise for training family therapists *Journal of Marital & Family Therapy, 27,* 535–544.

Irvine, J. L. (1992). Making teacher education culturally responsive. In *Diversity in teacher education,* M. E. Dilworth (ed.). San Francisco, CA: Jossey–Bass.

Kim, B. S. K., & Lyons, H. Z. (2003). Experiential activities and multicultural counseling competence training. *Journal of Counseling & Development, 81,* 400–408.

Leong, F. T. L., & Wagner, N. S. (1994). Cross–cultural counseling supervision: What do we know? What we need to know? *Counselor Education & Supervision, 34,* 117.

Miller, W. R., & Rollnick, S. (2002). *Motivational interviewing: Preparing people for change* (2nd ed.). New York, NY: Guiliford Press.

Minor, K. M. (1983). *A review of counseling among counselors with emphasis upon culture specific counseling within the Anent society: A method training program.* Unpublished docotoral dissertation, University of Massachusetts–Amherst, Amherst, MA.

National Council of La Raza (2008).*Fact sheet: The status of Latinos in the labor force.* Retrieved from http://www.nclr.org/content/publications/detail/50719/

Ortega, D. M., & Martinez, L. M. (2009). *The state of Latinos: Census 2010: Defining an agenda for the future.* New York, NY: Fundacion Azteca America.

Perez, S. M. (2004). Shaping new possibilities for Latino children and the nation's future. *Future of Children, 14*(2), 122–126.

Pew Hispanic Center (2006). *Statistical portrait of Hispanics in the United States.* Retrieved from www.pewhispanic.org/factsheets/factsheet.php?FactsheetID=35

Rae, W. A., & Willis, D. J. (1973). Effectiveness of discussion, modeling and experiential simulation in training empathy skills to medical students. Retrieved from ERIC.

Salazar, M., Bornstein-Gomez, M., Mercado, S., Martinez, L. M., Ortega, D. M., Somoza, O., Mendez, W., & Leon, A. (2008). *Agenda Latina: The state of Latinos 2008: Defining an agenda for the future.* Denver, CO: University of Denver Latino Center for Community Engagement and Scholarship.

Santiago-Rivera, A. L., Arredondo, P., & Gallardo-Cooper, M. (2002). *Counseling Latinos and La Familia: A practical guide* (vol. 17). Thousand Oaks, CA: Sage Publications.

Shepard, D. S. (2002). Innovative methods. *Counselor Education & Supervision, 42*, 145–158.

Suleiman, L. (2003). *Creating a Latino child welfare agenda: A strategic framework for change.* New York, NY: Committee for Hispanic Children and Families, Inc.

Torres Jr., S., & Ottens, A. J. (1997). The multicultural infusion process: A research–based approach. *Counselor Education & Supervision, 37*, 6–18.

Wehrmann, K. C., Shin, H., & Poertner, J. (2002). Transfer of training: An evaluation study. *Journal of Health & Social Policy, 15*(3/4), 23–37.

Wentz, R., & Gerber, N. (2009). *Training to change.* Retrieved from http://www.wentztraining.com

Zambrana, R. E., & Dorrington, C. (1998). Economic and social vulnerability of Latino children and families by subgroup: Implications for child welfare. *Child Welfare, 77*, 5–27.

Translating Knowledge for Child Welfare Practice Cross-Nationally

JULIE COOPER ALTMAN, GEMJOY BARRETT, JENISE BROWN,
LUVELLA CLARK-IDUSOGIE, YAMINAH MCCLENDON,
TANYA RUIZ, CHENELLE SKEPPLE, and LATARSHA THOMAS

Some researchers contend that the rise in child abuse allegations among Caribbean immigrants in New York City is consistent with the large body of research suggesting that maltreatment is driven by the complex interaction of interpersonal, economic, social, and environmental factors. Others believe it has more to do with cultural child-rearing norms sanctioning the use of physical punishment of children. The goals of the research reported here were to better understand the influence of these many factors on child rearing, particularly as they relate to disciplinary practices within the Trinidadian population. An ethnographic field study of the context and norms of child rearing in the Caribbean was completed. This yielded data that were then translated into practice guidelines and policy recommendations by seven seasoned child welfare workers in New York City, all involved in a specialized MSW training program with the principal investigator. The functioning of Caribbean immigrant families is affected by a combination of relocation issues, differing child-rearing norms and traditions, shifting family roles and parental expectations, economic hardships, and normative stressors. Knowledge of how better to address these in practice should aid in limiting their risk for family violence.

Public child welfare agencies across the United States have been profoundly influenced by recent demographic shifts. The fastest growing group of children living in our country today (one in five) is either foreign-born or the child of immigrants (Urban Institute, 2006; Hernandez, 2004). As more of these families become known to public child welfare, assessing these children's risk while supporting their caretakers' capacities to protect and nurture requires a more highly skilled and able child welfare workforce than ever before. Workers are needed who are respectful of diversity, receptive to specific cultural knowledge and differences, able to translate that knowledge into concrete, culturally competent strategies for practice and who can respond with a growing capacity for critical thinking and good judgment (Lincroft, Resner, Leung, & Bussiere, 2006; Velazquez, Vidal De Haymes, & Mindell, 2006; Molina, Garrett, & Monterio-Leitner, 2006; Pine & Drachman, 2005; Earner, 2005; Dettlaff & Rycraft, 2006).

This article reports on a unique research to practice project designed to increase the capacity of child welfare workers in these ways, to better serve immigrant Caribbean families. Development and translation of empirical knowledge about the context and norms of child-rearing in Trinidad for child welfare practice in the United States were jointly conducted by one faculty and seven MSW child welfare worker-student trainees. The collaborative project had as its objectives: 1) to increase the capacity child welfare workers have for culturally competent child welfare service delivery; 2) to develop a model of research to practice that could help child welfare workers process and use empirical data in their work; and 3) to increase the awareness and use of culturally appropriate, practical, responsive and effective child welfare practice and services available to immigrant families in the United States.

The research on which this article is based focused on understanding the context and norms of child-rearing among low-income, urban, Afro-Trinidadian families, many of whom have, or may, emigrate at some point to the United States. The original study goals were to: 1) better understand the historical, social, economic, ethnic and cultural contexts of child rearing in Trinidad and Tobago; 2) examine how these contexts determine norms of parenting, including nurturing, attachment, values transmission and disciplinary practices; and 3) propose culturally sensitive and appropriate interventions based on these findings that may better serve the growing population of Caribbean families in the U.S. child welfare system.

Ethnographic field data collected over a 6-month period from one community in the Caribbean highlights the multitude and complexity of children and family's needs as Trinidad and Tobago focuses on achieving "first world" status by 2020. Firsthand accounts of contemporary child rearing offered clear, contextual knowledge, which was then used to inform practice with families as they cycle in and out of the United States as transnational immigrants.

The need for further knowledge development and dissemination in the area of child welfare practice with Caribbean families in the United States is great. New York City, for example, is experiencing a dramatic increase in the numbers of immigrants (Fix & Capps, 2002). More than one third of its 8 million persons are foreign born, an "all-time high." Within these numbers is a significant increase in families with children (Chahine & van Straaten, 2005), many of whom may come to the attention of child welfare authorities (Figure 1).

Some researchers contend that the rise in child abuse allegations among Caribbean immigrants in New York City is consistent with the large body of research that suggests their functioning is affected by a combination of the kind of normative stressors all families experience in growing families and rearing children, as well as relocation issues such as adjusting to urban living, differing child rearing norms and traditions, shifting family roles and parental expectations, and economic hardships, placing them at higher risk for family violence and subsequent attention of public child welfare authorities (Dettlaff & Earner, 2007; Douglas-Hall & Koball, 2004; Segal & Maydas, 2005; Malley-Morrison, 2004; Carten, Rock, & Best-Cummings, 2002). Others believe it has more to do with cultural child–rearing norms sanctioning the use of physical punishment of children (Gopaul-McNicol, 1999; Payne, 1989; Arnold, 1982; Daniel, 2004), thus placing them at higher risk for protective service investigation (see Figure 2).

The goals of the research reported on here were to better understand the influence of current contextual factors on normative parenting patterns, particularly as they relate to disciplinary practices within the Trinidadian population. Then, using that knowledge, seven seasoned child welfare workers from the United States, all involved in a specialized MSW child welfare work-

---

I've been a public child welfare worker for over 12 years now, and have had many cases involving immigrant referrals. They frequently sound something like this: A Caribbean immigrant mother moves to the United States with her young child. The public school he attends reports excessive corporal punishment, and makes a Childline referral (child abuse and neglect report), as required by New York state law. The child alleges that his mother used a belt to discipline him after the school called last week reporting that the child was disrupting the class. During the protective service investigation, the mother confirms that she beat the child because as a child she was beaten and learned from the beating she received. The mother professes her belief that you whip a child because you love the child, though she admitted resenting the fact that she was beaten as a child. The mother usually works two jobs to provide for her family. She praises herself for having not left her child(ren) behind, like her own mother had done with her, leaving her at the mercy of abusive relatives back home. She claims that the child welfare worker has no understanding of the love she has for the child; her using corporal punishment now will spare the chance later in life that the police might beat or kill him. She believes that no one has the right to dictate the way she should raise her child.

FIGURE 1 GemJoy: A Typical Case.

New York is full of parents doing the best they can in an environment that can make their every effort difficult. There are so many influences that they can do little to limit. Their kids are exposed to all kinds of things that they wish they weren't, and the culture often appears to undermine their own parental authority. While trying to operate mostly under the radar of (ACS) child welfare authorities, their kids threaten them with reports to the very same!

FIGURE 2 Tanya: The Tug Between Immigrant Parents and their Children.

force training and retention program with the principal investigator, crafted a number of concrete, usable practice interventions and policies designed to better serve the growing population of Caribbean families who immigrate to the United States and become involved in the child welfare system.

What sets this contribution apart from others includes its unique transnational approach and a focus on contemporary, practical, usable knowledge. The empirical data the interventions are based on were derived from native, in vivo field research, yielding unparalleled insight into everyday parenting practices in the immigrants' home country, and grounded in its current socio-economic-political realities. The translation of this data into concrete, practical intervention and policy recommendations for immigrant child welfare services in the United States was done by experienced New York City-based child welfare professionals, who knew well the public child welfare context that the recommendations would have to fit.

METHODS

The primary research question posed in the initial, Caribbean-based, empirical investigation was, "What are the contemporary context and cultural norms in which children in one Trinidadian community are reared?" Full institutional review board approval from the primary author's home university was granted. Ethnographic data were collected over a 6-month period in a single, urban African-Trinidadian community, comprised largely of residents residing in a low-income public housing development adjacent to the capital city of Port-of-Spain and bordering the main highway of the country. The immigration pattern of families from this community is one of serial and sporadic transnationalism. A significant number of family members from this area live and/or work, at least part-time, in the United States (Figure 3).

Community Sample

The community in which the field research was conducted is made up mainly of nuclear family households, the majority of which include children. Of the

It's been my experience as a Child Protective Specialist employed with the city of New York that migrating families often relocate to busy congested neighborhoods and reside with immediate and extended relatives in overcrowded living conditions. These families live in substandard housing conditions, because the adult household members are frequently undocumented or are unable to afford adequate housing.

FIGURE 3 Yaminah: Risk in Residence.

households that comprise this community, 37% were headed by women alone. Families in the community were mainly Christian, with 75% of African descent and 19% of mixed race parentage. In 95% of households, at least one person had attended some secondary schooling; none had tertiary education. Approximately 43.5% had a family member employed in the formal sector, whereas 30% were unemployed and 26.5% self-employed. Most of the residents either rent (40%) or own (36%) their homes; 18% were squatting. Of the households in the community, 70% reported average incomes of less than US$500 per month, at least some coming from remittances from family members in the United States.

Data Collection

Ethnographic data collected as part of this study included multiple, extended interviews with randomly selected parents in this community using a semi-structured guide ($n = 28$); lengthy, multiple interviews with community children ($n = 42$), their teachers ($n = 8$), and other child-rearing "experts" ($n = 6$); semi-structured community observation including home visits and visits to schools and community agencies; and numerous drawings, artifacts, and photographs collected in the field. Parents and children of the community were randomly selected for observation and interview, and are representative, demographically, of the community's population. Child-rearing "experts" were identified using snowball sampling techniques, initiated by a key informant from a national parenting coalition. These experts included child advocates, parent trainers, social workers, and other government personnel responsible for parenting, youth, and family initiatives.

Trustworthiness

To enhance this study's validity, interviews were completed over a period of 6 months, in keeping with the standard of prolonged engagement with the community. They were tape recorded and transcribed. Extensive field notes and a reflexive journal were kept. Other analytic strategies used to increase trustworthiness included member checking, triangulation and use of an external auditor. Member checking was iterative, checking the fit of tentative codes or themes with participants on an ongoing basis as developed analytically from the data. Methodological triangulation was achieved in several ways: by interviewing parents, teachers and children of the community's school and by gathering narrative, observational and artifact kinds of data. External auditing was provided weekly by a key contact in Trinidad, a social worker with research experience who was also familiar with the community in which the study was conducted. Decisions with respect to data collection, coding, and analysis were processed with the social worker in Trinidad, enhancing openness and potential reproducibility.

Analysis

Qualitative data were coded and analyzed according to constant comparative method protocols. Numerous strategies to visually display and organize the data were also applied. Quantitative data were coded and appropriate statistical analyses of these data were conducted using SPSS (SPSS Version 14.0, SPSS, Inc., Chicago, IL).

RESULTS

Context is defined here as the interrelated conditions in which child rearing exists or is concerned with. *Norms* are considered to be the ideal standards binding the members of a group and serving to guide, control, or regulate proper and acceptable or customary parenting and/or child-rearing behavior. The contextual factors found to undergird child-rearing in the Caribbean are inextricably interwoven and include historical, religious or moral, economic, political, social, cultural, and global influences (see Figures 4 and 5).

Contextual Factors

Findings regarding the context of child rearing in Trinidad yielded a number of themes, the most predominant being the importance of physical discipline and corporal punishment in normative child rearing. Historically, physical

---

As a child welfare worker, I have observed a significant number of factors that contribute to a family becoming involved with the local child welfare agency. Some of these factors may stem from the culture of the country of origin, while other factors are the result of trying to navigate the new (American) culture. Working with a family that is unaware of the role of a child welfare agency is difficult.

FIGURE 4 Latarsha: Assimilation and Acculturation.

In my experience, families have too often been scared to death to ask for the kind of help that may have prevented the very problem I am investigating them for! But I understand it ... some of them think they will be deported if they become known to government organizations like HRA or ACS; some of them worry what their relatives will think of them needing assistance here in this great land of plenty. I think others just can't imagine ever being put in the position where things have gotten so out of control for them and their families ... they can't even admit it to themselves.

FIGURE 5 Luvella: Implications of Seeking Help.

punishment was used to strengthen and police the patriarchal/authoritarian hierarchies during colonial and post-colonial periods, a pattern that continues privately today. Entrenched notions of physical discipline as love and safety remain, often seen by residents as "good for us." Community members frequently made statements such as "If he hits me, he loves me," or a similar phrase. The "spare the rod, spoil the child" mantra was heard extensively with parents taking seriously the need to teach children right from wrong, not merely to curb bad behavior (see Figure 6). The pervasive influence and acceptance of the use of physical force in child rearing was seen in both historical and popular culture, including rhymes and games played by children. Recent growth in conservative Protestantism in the Caribbean reinforces this ethic.

Political and economic forces found to impact patterns of child rearing were significant. Children in the community studied are now the second generation of "structurally adjusted poor." The economic security fears and anxieties that poor parents experience as they try to provide for their families grows daily, as they are disproportionately burdened by new political and global realities. Trinidad and Tobago's race to attain "First World" status by 2020 finds workers being wooed by incentive pay for longer and weekend working hours, while often facing 3- to 4-hour daily commutes (using infrastructure not meant to sustain the growing capacity of cars and residents).

I have worked with many parents who report problems in adjusting to "American" child rearing norms something like this: "Taking away privileges, being told to put my child in his room as punishment, this was anathema to me as a Caribbean mother rearing a child in this country. That took him away from engaging with me, and it didn't work! I've had to fully reconsider ways that allow interaction between the two of us, which I consider crucial to his getting the messages that I care for him and I want him to learn, but that don't go over the edge into what would be considered here as 'abusive'."

FIGURE 6 Chenelle: A Cultural Child Rearing Conundrum.

Those unable to find work due to recent economic conditions follow long entrenched patterns of seasonal or full-time migration, usually led by one or more adults of the extended family.

The contemporary social problem found most stressful for parents is an increasingly high violent crime rate, leading to fears for personal safety, increased social isolation, less use of traditionally effective "community minding" of children, and existential concerns about what role parents and other community citizens are seen to play in the propagation of violence. A spiritual longing was also expressed by many families, as they witness the replacement of genuine love toward children and time spent with children by material items. In addition, while the media imports more examples of parenting skills and discipline to consider, these imports are models with outcomes (i.e., spoiled children) that parents report not wishing to replicate. Soaring AIDS rates lead to national questions about trust—who can I trust, even in my own family? Greater migration of extended family members, combined with the AIDS crisis, limit the number of healthy, available adults who might be available for child minding or child shifting (moving children to live with other family members or friends temporarily), long-resilient strategies for the healthy rearing of children in this community and many Caribbean communities.

Child-Rearing Norms

The twin ethics of respectability and reputation as well as a strong sense of accountability and close behavioral control of children undergird contemporary child rearing norms. Respect from children is highly valued, as is public appearance and direct obedience. The idea of children as property of which to be proud leads to a strong sense of accountability because families believe it is both their right and responsibility to rear children without government interference. Parents expressed a lot of fear and discomfort in giving children any kind of choice or decision-making power, rejecting the notion that discipline should build individual problem-solving capacities in children. Also rejected, largely, is the idea that parent–child relationships, communication, positive reinforcement and nurturing might replace the need for punishment, often espoused in Western, developed-country models of positive parenting and preventive discipline.

A number of child-rearing practices in this community can be seen as normative risk factors for the children of this community: a lack of a parent–child relationship, many examples of parenting by fear, tremendous emphasis on school achievement, prevalent over- or under-disciplining, a dearth of ways in which love can be legitimately and safely shown, great disdain for state oversight/interference, and implicit notions or experiences of corporal punishment among most family members ("*corporal punishment didn't hurt me, so ...*"). The soon-to-be-enacted Trinidad and Tobago Children's Act, institutionalizing public child welfare, protective services, and normative standards of community child-rearing, was embraced by experts, but resisted by most community members, whose fear that their capacity to rear children privately and "rightly" will be severely limited.

Summary of Findings

In sum, what was found were that children's needs in this Caribbean community were greater than that of earlier generations, given the socioeconomic and political context and social/cultural realities, requiring more, not less, discipline and nurturing. Parents and community members all referred to greater numbers of "harden[ed]" (stubborn and recalcitrant) children in their community. Parents' anxiety and confusion about what is happening in society and with their children lead to inappropriate use of fewer alternatives of child-rearing and child discipline, poor role modeling, and fear of a power imbalance in the family. Community norms and supports are changing rapidly, with relationships, trust, voice, and power all in a state of flux. Further, the view that corporal punishment is not, nor is it related to, child abuse and neglect is pervasive, despite what the United Nations Convention on the Rights of the Child states (of which Trinidad and Tobago and many other Caribbean and developing countries were early signatories). And, given that 75% of social work students at the University of the West Indies (St. Augustine, Trinidad) endorsed corporal punishment as an effective means of child-rearing, this practice is likely to remain a durable one (Altman, 2007).

TRANSLATING KNOWLEDGE TO PRACTICE AND POLICY

The initial idea of using these findings to promote better child welfare practice began at a farewell breakfast meeting attended by the primary author with some students prior to the author's sabbatical as a Fulbright Scholar to the University of the West Indies in Trinidad and Tobago. The students were MSW trainees, part of a federally funded child welfare workforce retention project directed by the primary author. Their idea was seen as having twofold benefits: 1) to maintain ties with their professor during sabbatical and reap further educational benefits related to that experience, and 2) to use what they learned to formulate and promote better practice strategies to immigrant families in New York City's public child welfare system, where all of them remained employed as protective service workers. A plan to achieve these aims was developed at that breakfast, and carried out over the 6 months their professor was in Trinidad and Tobago.

Background literature, excerpts from field notes and periodic analytic memos based on primary data were sent periodically from the primary investigator to the students back in the United States by electronic mail during the first 5 months of the project. Findings (as noted previously) were shared electronically several weeks prior to the students' arrival in Trinidad for a 1-week stay. Extensive electronic mail and phone communication occurred in preparation for this in-country experience. On arrival of the worker-student trainees in Trinidad, a number of long discussions of the empirical study's findings were held. Analytic processes continued, with each student then focusing on developing one particular area from the findings, articulating potential practice innovations, policy changes, and organizational responses.

Practice Innovations

A number of practice strategies were developed, informed by the empirical knowledge gained in-country but articulated by the U.S. child welfare workers on the research team. These strategies included holding focused conversations with clients regarding discipline, corporal punishment, the nature of government-sponsored child welfare services, their children, fears, and expectations; affirmation of parenting strengths pre-migration; emphasis of development of social networks and skills related to community-building; and development of practical strategies of acceptable punishment. It is understood that many of these strategies may only be implemented following appropriate worker training and then only with proper support and follow-through by supervisors and managers, as with most practice innovations in child welfare.

Focused conversations were conceptualized to be productive dialogues that may help child welfare workers better understand cognitive and contextual underpinnings of the parenting behavior in question. These conversations could stimulate a plethora of potential targets for education, alternative parenting strategies, support, or the offering of other appropriate intervention or resources. Ideally these discussions could include the meaning and consequences physical discipline has for them and the child socially, culturally and spiritually, its anticipated and real outcomes, and their awareness and understanding of alternative techniques. For example, workers could fully explore the meaning parents place on corporal punishment, their sense of its usefulness, its effectiveness, its purpose, and its outcome for both them as parents as for their children.

By exploring the family's notions of why they feel the need to use corporal punishment, and how they see it working for them, child welfare workers may more collaboratively work to seek a common understanding of a family's frequent dilemma. They want the child to feel loved and cared for, but also want to stay clear of state interference. These explorations may also help to forge a mutual relationship, without imposing judgment on a valued (and seen to be effective) child-rearing practice. Discussing with the family the various alternatives to corporal punishment they may have tried, and with what results, may also be fruitful. Asking what alternatives they may consider using could reinforce their initiative, instead of imposing from a power position.

Altering, not eliminating, the practice of corporal punishment may be appropriately suggested. Having others inflict the punishment, for example, may limit the potential for bodily harm that may come with punishment given in anger or frustration. Waiting for the rage to subside before inflicting punishment could also be a strategy that may work—counting to 10, for example, or eating a piece of fruit before the punishment is administered. These practical strategies, designed to increase the probability of use of acceptable punishment in immigrant families, many of whom equate physical means with love and caring, were seen to be relatively easy to implement and low cost.

Conversations which draw on what immigrant parents may have seen as their parenting strengths pre-migration was seen as another helpful strengths-based strategy to try. Child welfare workers can ask what they hope and dream for their children in this new country, what they fear for their child or themselves, and what differences they or their children have had to adjust to. Conversations around what their children were like when they left the Caribbean or other home country and what they are like now could also yield helpful data to plan interventions around. These discussions may help workers in assessing the skills and capacities these parents have or may need to expand upon in order for new strategies to succeed. Patience, communication, and the ability to delay gratification can all better be assessed through extended, meaningful conversations within the family.

Working to better understand their notions of the institution of child welfare in the United States and how they see the role of the state in the private lives of families may also lead to a fruitful discussion of differences and misunderstandings. Many Caribbean families are fearful of the large police presence they view in New York City compared with their home countries, particularly given the extreme violence many have been exposed to in their home countries coupled with their disdain for authority. Exploring these fears and communicating about differing standards of civil and social control may lead to fruitful discussions about the rights and responsibilities of families and community residents.

Similarly, questions of how affiliated they are with the Caribbean community in the United States, the type of support network they have, and where they go for the resources they need should be addressed with immigrant families. Understanding the dynamics of the family's social ties, relationships, and roles may help identify specific burdens and stressors that have contributed to concerns about a child's welfare or well-being. In addition, it may help bring competencies and personal and social strengths to the surface that the client had not previously realized were present. For many new immigrants, social networks are key to their being able to thrive in the United States and help to fortify against the erosion of the once valuable community child-minding many are experiencing in the Caribbean.

Policy Innovations

Policy changes, based on knowledge gained from the field research reported on earlier in this article, were also identified and recommended by the research team. These changes could have profound effects on the capacity Caribbean immigrants have to rear their children here in the US One such innovation is getting information to newly arriving parents regarding the laws and norms of child-rearing in the United States in order to clear up miscommunication, allay fears, and, hopefully, enlarge the repertoire of acceptable child-rearing strategies parents can legitimately and safely choose from once living in the United States. Newcomers should at the same time be given information on other child and family supportive agencies and services, where they may find help proactively should family issues arise. Other policy innovations are those better suited for community social workers, policy practitioners, schools of social work and other large social institutions to carry out, targeting mezzo and macro level impacts. These include community development and growth, changes in U.S. immigration and economic policies, and combating the persistent negative influence of racism. Advocacy and social action strategies to reduce these system level risk factors, taught in Schools of Social Work as Council on Social Work Education mandated core competencies, can have broad impact.

Migrating families are often profoundly and disproportionately affected by economic risk factors. Some of the variables that contribute to these families' vulnerability for child abuse and neglect reporting are economic hardship, large household size, substandard housing, and unemployment or underemployment at low wage jobs. For migrating families, financial responsibility rests largely on the head of household. In Caribbean families, head of household is often the mother, and the ability to effectively provide for their family, while being responsible for most of the burden of child rearing and child minding, can become overwhelming. Oftentimes, the primary caretaker obtains several employments to maintain the needs of their immediate family members and supplement income for their extended household and families abroad, sometimes jobs that keep them away from their family throughout the week.

Serial migration of families from the Caribbean has also been an adaptive strategy for coping with future familial and economic uncertainties for many years. West Indians, in particular, see keeping a transnational identity as a strategy for place-holding in the socioeconomic hierarchy. To be seen as "American"—which for many from the Caribbean once they arrive here means to be seen as African American—leads to downward social mobility. Instead, they often strengthen and broaden their transnational links and networks, increasingly easy given their geography, low airfare, the internet, and other inexpensive telecommunications. While transnational ties have many benefits, they may also serve to increase rather than decrease the stress of migration.

Advocating for more equitable, fair, socially just immigration, and global economic policies, such as living wages, can do much to influence these needs. Advocacy is taught as part of the repertoire of skills all good social workers (and citizens) have at their disposal no matter their auspices. The National Association of Social Workers (Washington, DC), social agencies, and schools of social work can be pressed to emphasize the impact, importance, and ethical nature of this social change obligation.

Education about how U.S. markets and consumer behavior directly affect the finances and economic burdens of families, particularly in developing nations, is needed in all levels of higher education, but particularly in schools of social work. Policy can help that directly affects the global economic conditions that many West Indians and other immigrants from developing countries face, so that the billions of dollars of remittances annually sent back to extended families can be redirected toward improving the economic conditions of the immigrants themselves.

Social action that continues to chip away at the pervasive effects of racism in the United States will also impact these socioeconomic conditions with which many West Indian immigrants, and African-Americans overall, struggle. *Erase Racism* (Syosset, NY), and other similar organizations providing education, awareness, and advocacy around racial inequality, should be supported by schools of social work and social work agencies, including the public child welfare agencies, through encouraging and funding training and workshops for their students/personnel.

A more pragmatic policy strategy is providing information to immigrants before they migrate to the United States. The time of a protective services investigation is not the optimal time to inform an immigrant family of child welfare practices in the host country. A comprehensive awareness plan would seek to inform newly arriving parents of the laws of the United States with respect to parental rights and obligations, the norms of US child-rearing, including age-appropriate guidelines of self-care and supervised care, acceptable strategies and techniques of discipline, an overview of the child welfare system in the United States, and a resource list of child- and family-oriented agencies and websites that could help to support them. Plans are underway to develop a brochure in conjunction with the U.S. Embassy in Trinidad and Tobago (Figure 7).

For more than eight years, I have been a child welfare investigator. Over the years I have come in contact with more immigrant families. These families are often unaware of the laws regarding child protection and are only made aware of such laws at the time that they are the subject of a child abuse/neglect investigation. In an effort to provide the most appropriate and comprehensive services to these families, it is important to educate the family prior to becoming involved with the child welfare system.

FIGURE 7 Jenise: Immigrant Awareness of Child Welfare.

DISCUSSION

Findings reported here with respect to the influence of historical, religious, social, cultural, and global factors on family structure and child rearing in the Caribbean are similar to those emphasized in others' work (Adams, 2000; Daniel, 2004; Gopaul McNichol, 1999; Payne, 1989). The durability of these findings is striking and poses a significant dilemma to the child welfare practitioner who too often views the child and/or family in a narrow, secular context without due attention to the influence of these important mores (Matthews & Mahoney, 2005). Denying immigrant parents the option of corporal punishment of their children in the United States, for example, could be seen as ineffective at best, serving to exacerbate behaviors and dynamics that could ironically lead to a greater likelihood of more significant abuse, at worst. Focused conversations that bring out these hidden concerns are recommended as well as other practical interpersonal strategies designed to support parents in child rearing.

Political and economic forces found to affect patterns of child rearing for both native Trinidadians and those who emigrate were somewhat different than those articulated in past research (Girvan, 1997; Ayeni, Reif, & Thomas, 2000). Increasing rates of violence, eroding community norms, and political emphasis on achieving "first world" status have substantially affected child rearing in unanticipated ways, influencing not only rates of emigration but also the needs of the families once they arrive. Macro-level policy and practice recommendations made here can yield broad-based change and include social action, community development, advocacy, and economic policy development strategies.

Improving the capacity of child welfare workers to deliver culturally competent and effective services builds on the commitment of many who have pioneered this kind of translation work (Carten & Goodman, 2005; Pine & Drachman, 2005; Earner & Rivera, 2005). The translation of knowledge gained from a study such as this, considering evidence on the context and norms of child-rearing in Trinidad and turning it into strategies for effective, culturally sensitive, and appropriate child welfare practice in New York City, not only yields better service for the growing population of Caribbean families in the child welfare system but also increased capacity of these and other workers to do similar translation for other immigrant groups. As more extraordinarily diverse families come to the attention of the public child welfare system, direct service workers will need these and similar skills (Altman & Michael, 2007). Preparing and delivering services that are culturally syntonic with the needs of all immigrant populations remains an important social work priority and a promising area of new knowledge development (Dettlaff, 2008; Drachman & Paulino, 2004; Russell & White, 2001; Fong, 2004).

SUMMARY AND CONCLUSIONS

The work described here aims to have an impact on social work education for the professionalization of the child welfare workforce and child welfare practice at a number of levels. First, models such as the one presented here or similar but modified versions may be models that other schools can replicate in training child welfare workers. Such unique training experiences can serve to assist future student social workers in gaining skills necessary for translating empirical evidence into good field practice, generally, while at the same time helping them to learn practical strategies as they interface increasingly with immigrant families in the child welfare system, specifically.

Second, the empirical, field-based findings presented here about the norms and contexts of child-rearing in the Caribbean are disseminated with the hope that readers might translate them for their own practice and policy in the public child welfare context with similar or different immigrant populations. Child welfare professionals will increasingly be asked to develop critical skills in translating the growing empirical knowledge base into professional practice (Kessler, Gira & Poertner, 2005; Mederos & Woldeguiorguis, 2003; Miller & Gaston, 2003).

Finally, it is hoped that some readers may also find ways to integrate some of the practice and policy innovations suggested here directly into their current child welfare practice and organizational contexts. In this evidence-based world, workers should continue to challenge themselves to incorporate empirically based knowledge as part of good critical thinking processes and practice.

REFERENCES

Adams, C. J. (2000). Integrating children into families separated by migration: A Caribbean–American case study. *Journal of Social Distress and the Homeless,* *9*(1), 19–27.

Altman, J. C. (2007, October). *Toward understanding the durability of the use of corporal punishment among Trinidadians*. Paper presented at the 2nd Caribbean Research Conference on Children's Issues, Kingston, Jamaica.

Altman, J. C., & Michael, S. (2007). Exploring the immigrant experience: An empirically-based tool for practice in child welfare. *Protecting Children, 22*(2), 42–54.

Arnold, E. (1982). The use of corporal punishment in child rearing in the West Indies. *Child Abuse and Neglect, 6*, 2, 141–145.

Ayeni, V., Reif, L. & Thomas, H. (2000). *Strengthening ombudsman and human rights institutions in commonwealth small and island states: The Caribbean experience*. London, England: Commonwealth Secretariat.

Carten, A., & Goodman, H. (2005). An educational model for child welfare practice with English-speaking Caribbean families. *Child Welfare, 84*, 771–789.

Carten, A., Rock, L. & Best-Cummings, C. (2002). Dimensions of abuse and neglect among native and immigrant Caribbean families. *Journal of Immigrant and Refugee Services, 1*(2), 41–57.

Chahine, Z., & van Straaten, J. (2005). Serving immigrant families and children in New York City's child welfare system. *Child Welfare, 84*, 713–723.

Daniel, C. A. (2004). Social work with West Indian families: A multilevel approach. *Journal of Immigrant and Refugee Services, 2*, 135–145.

Dettlaff, A. J. (2008). Immigrant Latino children and families in child welfare: A framework for conducting a cultural assessment. *Journal of Pubic Child Welfare, 2*, 451–470.

Dettlaff, A. J., & Earner, I. (Eds.). (2007). The intersection of migration and child welfare: Emerging issues and implications [special issue]. *Protecting Children, 22*, 2.

Dettlaff, A. J., & Rycraft, J. R. (2006). The impact of migration and acculturation on Latino children and families: Implications for child welfare practices. *Protecting Children, 21*, 6–21.

Douglas-Hall, A., & Koball, H. (2004). *Children of recent immigrants: National and regional trends*. New York, NY: National Center for Children in Poverty.

Drachman, D., & Paulino, A. (2004). *Immigrants and social work: Thinking beyond the borders of the United States*. Binghamton, NY: Haworth.

Earner, I. (2005). Immigrant children and youth in the child welfare system. In G. Mallon & P. Hess (Eds.), *Child welfare for the twenty-first century: A handbook of practices, policies and programs* (pp. 655–664). New York, NY: Columbia.

Earner, I., & Rivera, H. (2005). Special issue: Immigrants and refugees and child welfare. *Child Welfare, 84*, 1–5.

Fix, M. E., & Capps, R. (2002). *The dispersal of immigrants in the 1990s*. Washington, DC: The Urban Institute.

Fong, R. (2004). Contexts and environments for culturally competent practice. In R. Fong (Ed.), *Culturally competent practice with immigrant and refugee children and families* (pp. 38–59). New York, NY: Guilford.

Girvan, N. (Ed.) (1997). Poverty, empowerment and social development in the Caribbean. Kingston, Jamaica: Consortium Graduate School of Social Sciences.

Gopaul-McNicol, S. A. (1999). Ethnocultural perspectives on childrearing practices in the Caribbean, *International Social Work, 42*(1), 79–86.

Hernandez, D. J. (2004). Demographic change and life circumstances of immigrant families. *The Future of Children, 14*, 17–47.

Kessler, M. L., Gira, E., & Poertner, J. (2005). Moving best practice to evidence-based practices in child welfare. *Families in Society, 86*, 244–250.

Lincroft, Y., Resner, J., Leung, M., & Bussiere, A. (2006). *Undercounted. Underserved. Immigrant and refugee families in the child welfare system.* Baltimore, MD: Annie E. Casey Foundation.

Matthews, L., & Mahoney, A. (2005). Facilitating a smooth transitional process for immigrant Caribbean children: The role of teachers, social workers, and related professional staff. *Journal of Ethnic and Cultural Diversity in Social Work, 14*(1/2), 69–92.

Malley-Morrison, K. (Ed.) (2004). *International perspectives on family violence and abuse: A cognitive ecological approach.* Mahwah, NJ: Erlbaum.

Mederos, E., & Woldeguiorguis, I. (2003). Beyond cultural competence: What child protection managers need to know and do. *Child Welfare, 82*, 125–142.

Miller, O. A., & Gaston, R. J. (2003). A model of culture-centered child welfare practice. *Child Welfare, 82*, 235–250.

Molina, B., Garrett, M. T., & Monterio-Leitner, J. (2006). Communities of courage: Caring for immigrant children and families through creative. *Protecting Children, 21*(2), 62–83.

Payne, M. A. (1989). Use and abuse of corporal punishment: a Caribbean view. *Child Abuse and Neglect, 13*, 389–401.

Pine, B. A., & Drachman, D. (2005). Effective child welfare practice with immigrant and refugee children and their families. *Child Welfare, 84*, 537–562.

Russell, M., & White, B. (2001). Practice with immigrants and refugees: Social work and client perspectives. *Journal of Ethnic and Cultural Diversity in Social Work, 9*, 73–92.

Segal, U. A., & Mayadas, N. S. (2005). Assessment of issues facing immigrant and refugee families. *Child Welfare, 84*, 563–583.

Urban Institute. (2006). *Children of immigrants: Facts and figures.* Washington, DC: Author. Retrieved from www.urban.org

Velazquez, S., Vidal de Haymes, M., & Mindell, R. (2006). Migration: A critical issue for child welfare. *Protecting Children, 21*, 2–4.

An Empirically Based Field-Education Model: Preparing Students for Culturally Competent Practice with New Immigrants

ALMA J. CARTEN
and
JEANNE BERTRAND FINCH

This article reports implementation themes and a content analysis of student portfolios and learning contracts from year one of a 4-year service/educational initiative undertaken with metropolitan schools of social work, the public child welfare agency, and community-based agencies serving new immigrants. The initiative designed, implemented and evaluated a model preparing MSW students for culturally competent preventive practice with immigrant families. The discussion identifies: emerging themes, implications, and the challenges and benefits of university–public child welfare collaborations in addressing the needs of immigrant children and their families.

This article reports the first-year findings of a 4-year initiative implemented in partnership with schools of social work, the public child welfare agency, and community-based agencies. The Immigrant Child Welfare Project (ICWFP) was undertaken in response to the influx of new immigrants from Mexico and Latin American, Central American, and West African countries, and their corresponding increase on child welfare caseloads. The initiative designed, implemented, and evaluated educational/service models preparing MSW students for culturally competent practice with target immigrant populations. The discussion identifies emerging themes for continued model building; and encourages university–public collaborations in preparing social work students for child welfare practice in an increasingly global environmental context.

BACKGROUND

Changing demographics of the child welfare caseload, legislative priorities of the 1997 Adoptions and Safe Families Act (ASFA) and renewed partnerships among schools of social work and public child welfare agencies to improve child welfare outcomes through workforce development are among the contemporary trends that provided the rationale and design of the ICWFP. The ICWFP builds on findings from a study recommending specialized field practica to improve educational outcomes for Children's Services employees enrolled in MSW programs (Carten & Finch 1998), and replicates best practices from a pilot program targeting Anglo Caribbean immigrant families (Carten & Goodman, 2005).

Caseload trend data from New York City Children's Services' Division for Immigrant Services reveal growing linguistic diversity among families. According to these data, there are more than 40 languages and dialects spoken by families using child welfare services. Spanish is the most frequent request made by staff for language interpreters, and Mexicans are the fastest growing segment of Spanish speaking new immigrants. Further, the newest immigrants are increasingly from non-European countries, more culturally and linguistically diverse (Passel & Suro, 2005; Salvo, 2005) and more likely to experience discrimination related to race and ethnicity (Frances, 2000; Lincroft, Resner, Leung, & Bussiere, 2006). Further, new immigrants have low income, lack health insurance, and are food insecure (Capps, 1999; Urban Institute, 2002). Limited English skills and restricted access to government income and family support services place them at increased risk for poverty, one of the strongest predictors for child welfare involvement.

Concurrent with increasing diversity of the child welfare caseload, are redirections in child welfare policy encouraging the use of preventive community-based family support services to keep children safe in their own families and neighborhoods. Children's Services has incorporated legislative mandates into a reform plan that shifts emphasis from out-of-home care to a locally based system of care, and outcome-based practice approaches (Administration for Children's Services [ACS], 2007). A priority of the realignment plan is building community collaboratives with voluntary agencies committed to changing community conditions that place children at risk (Mattingly, 2005). The plan incorporates strategies that establish links with the immigrant advocate community and comprehensive plans for complying with legal mandates prohibiting discrimination based on national origin, language or immigration status (Chahine & van Stratten, 2005).

Each of these developments has reciprocal implications for schools of social work as they prepare new graduates for child welfare practice, and call for strengthening traditional alliances between schools of social work and public child welfare agencies. These partnerships provide organizational supports needed to develop innovative educational strategies that promote best practices for evidence-based, culturally competent interventions.

LITERATURE REVIEW

Educating for today's increasingly global practice context requires promotion of cultural sensitivity as the foundation for child welfare practice. Cultural competency is therefore an integrating theme of the ICWFP.

Since 1971, the Council on Social Work Education (CSWE) Curriculum Policy Statement has been consistently modified to ensure appropriate avenues of curriculum renewal and expanded definitions to keep pace with evolving diversity issues (CSWE, 2003). The National Association of Social Workers Standards for Cultural Competence (NASW, 2001), describe cultural competency as an ongoing process and identify elements that should be present at all levels of service delivery. Over the past decade, the Child Welfare League of America has made significant contributions to articulating culturally competent standards for best practice in child welfare settings at the organizational, systemic and practitioner levels (Nash & Velazquez, 2003). In response to the increasing linguistic and ethnic diversity of worker caseloads, Children's Services has instituted new initiatives that expand diversity dialogues in an effort to improve access to culturally and linguistically competent family support services for immigrant children (Chahine & van Stratten, 2005).

In addition to standards established by the aforementioned organizations, faculty scholarship has contributed to the discourse around culturally competent child welfare practice, and the extent to which this has been achieved and integrated in current practice (Balgopal, 2000; Belanger, Bullard & Green, 2008; Browne & Mills, 2001; Carten & Dumpson, 2004; Everett, Chipungu, & Leashore, 2004; Hill, 2006; Lum & Lu, 2007; McRoy, 2000; Roberts, 2002; Samantrai, 2004). Recent years also have seen an increase in faculty scholarship on culturally and linguistically competent practices with immigrant families (Balgopal, 2000; Carten & Goodman, 2005; Earner & Riviera, 2005; Furuto, 2004; Potocky-Trippodi, 2002; Pine & Drachman, 2005).

This literature underscores that best practices with immigrants require a mix of services addressing concrete services and mental health needs.

Additionally, a number of unique stressors related to the immigration experience contribute to increased needs for culturally competent mental health services (Balgopal, 2000; Drachman, 1992; Potocky-Tripodi, 2002). In addition to these increased needs is the need to emphasize institutional change approaches, to incorporate culturally appropriate practice strategies and interactional styles, and to respect for culturally based perspectives (Devore & Schlesinger, 1996; Potocky-Tripodi, 2002). Fellin (2000) encourages social work educators to continue the dialogue around multiculturalism in social work education and to revisit teaching multicultural practice in the context of dramatic demographic changes occurring in the United States. This process is critical for social work educators to contribute more fully in preparing students for culturally competent practice and in creating multicultural human service organizations and service delivery models. The ICWFP provides one example of this effort.

The ICWFP draws upon the substantial growth in practice and research literature that lends new insights into problems, service needs and help-seeking behaviors of diverse immigrant populations. Themes emerging from the targeted literature review have relevance for culturally competent child welfare practice with target immigrant populations and were integral in shaping the ICWFP design.

PROJECT DESCRIPTION

The Educational Model

The centerpiece of the ICWFP educational model is a specialized field-education unit located in community-based sites that are popular resettlement neighborhoods for new immigrant families. The units were structured to include a *school-based unit* in an elementary public school and an *agency-based unit* in a Children's Services' Division of a Child Protection Field Office. A *hospital-based unit*, in a municipal hospital serving a catchment area corresponding to those areas of the other two units, was added to improve case finding. Students are assigned to a designated field instructor and are responsible for providing a comprehensive array of services to target immigrant families.

Goals, Objectives, and Practice Principals

The ICWFP's goals are to develop, implement and evaluate an innovative educational model to prepare MSW students capable of providing culturally competent services to target immigrant families consistent with Children's Services' neighborhood-based model and ASFA priorities of safety, permanency, and child and family well-being. These goals are achieved through core educational and programmatic strategies of leadership development; enhanced educational programs that include intersession courses on child welfare and monthly clinical conferences; collaborative agency partnerships in the catchment areas; curriculum development for new electives and infusion into Children's Services in-service trainings; and utilization of the project's mixed research design to generate evidenced-based culturally competent practice. The conceptual design of the ICWFP is anchored in practice principals organized around concepts of the ecological perspective; strengths-based and empowerment approaches; dual concerns for child safety and preserving families; community as the base for service delivery; inclusion of stakeholders in administrative decision-making; and social capital development.

THE EVALUATION DESIGN

The mixed methods research design includes a survey of graduates; Pre–Post Test of Student Self-Reported Level of Multicultural Knowledge and Awareness (Ponterroto, Gretchen, Utsey, Riger, & Austin, 2002); content analysis of student materials and parent seminars; and the first year impact study. The findings reported here focus on materials obtained from the first-year cohort excluding the pre- and post-test of student self-reported level of multicultural knowledge and awareness and the survey of graduates. The pre–post multicultural knowledge and awareness self-assessment student scores are excluded due to insufficient numbers of students from this first-year cohort.

Reported qualitative measures include: student assessments of the educational enhancements, and themes emerging from student portfolios, learning contracts and seminar sessions for parents. Utilizing content analysis (Franzosi, 2008) of student portfolios and learning contracts provides a rich source of data related to the goals of the project. The analysis supports the evidenced-based component of the research design and identifies themes at three intervals during the academic year to assess knowledge, skills, and values to support competencies required for effective practice with immigrant families. The analysis also identifies themes about help-seeking and service utilization behaviors of target immigrant populations.

As the process evaluation is ongoing, it provides feedback for modifications at various stages of implementation (ICWFP 2006–2007 Implementation Report, 2008). Future reports will utilize quantitative findings of the integration of learning objectives of the program, the number of graduates continuing to practice in child welfare settings, the number of new courses relevant to child welfare practice with immigrant families offered at the participating Consortium schools, the pre- and post-self-reported level of multicultural knowledge and awareness scores and the first self-efficacy survey of graduates (Holden, Meenaghan, Anastas, & Metrey, 2002).

LIMITATIONS

The following interrelated problems of implementation impacted year-one goal achievement: the structure of communication channels did not fully support consensus building around the conceptual design of the educational model among all participating organizations; limited knowledge about target immigration groups at start-up slowed the process of engaging families and the development of full caseloads for all students; and the lack of case materials needed to support university requirements impacted the morale of some students. These factors created the climate within which students compiled their student portfolios and learning contracts, which were a primary source of data collection. Despite limitations, useful information regarding necessary supports to enhance student learning and cultural knowledge and awareness emerged. Although generalizations of findings are limited, identified themes have potential broad application and provide useful guides for further enquiry and model building.

Description of Participating Students

Thirteen students, representing seven schools of social work comprised the 2006–2007 cohort. Seven of the students were selected from Children's Services Professional Development Program and six from the general enrollment of the participating schools. Of the total number of students ($N = 13$), most students were female ($n = 11$). With the exception of one student, students were in their second year and enrolled in direct service concentrations. Three were first generation immigrants from Vietnam, Japan, and Nigeria. Six were first or second generation immigrants from the Anglo Caribbean, the Dominican Republic, and Latin and Central American countries. Two of the American-born students were African American, and two were Caucasian. Languages spoken included: English, Spanish, French, Japanese, Vietnamese, Chinese and an African dialect.

Description of Participant Families

Families served by the school-based unit were largely from French-speaking West African countries, including the Ivory Coast, Yemen, Mali, Senegal, and Sierra Leone. Families served by the agency-based unit included Mexican, Latin and Central American immigrants. A small number of families were from China, Vietnam, Bangladesh and the Anglo Caribbean. Families served within the hospital-based unit were from West Africa, Mexico, and Latin and Central America.

A large share of the West African immigrant families was Muslim. Key informants and project cultural guides indentified to assist with client engagement suggested that these families tended to be employed, with fathers working as taxi or livery drivers, and mothers in hair-braiding and craft shops. Some had earned professional degrees in their native countries that were not valid in the United States. Others held high status and prestige in their native countries because of family lineage or governmental and political appointments. Some left their homelands because of political turmoil others chose to leave to improve their economic situations. While extended kin of some continued to live in continental Africa; others were living abroad in the United Kingdom, France, and Canada. The heterogeneity amongst families' countries of national origin served by the agency-based unit, and challenges of case finding in year one limited our understanding of the specific characteristics of Hispanic families from Mexico and Latin and Central America.

RESULTS

The Parent Seminars

Monthly parent seminars conducted over the spring semester were among the mix of services provided. These seminars were co-facilitated by students with an expert consultant, and structured around ICWFP principles of empowerment and inclusion. These principles involved learning directly from parents which services they deemed critical for supporting families in the resettlement process. Topics covered focused on the participants' informational needs and used a didactic approach. Content included immigrant rights to entitlement programs, and policies essential for negotiating and accessing services provided by Children's Services and the Department of Education, Health and Housing. Other sessions were more interactive and examined stressors of the immigrant experience that had implications for family stability and child safety. Topical themes of these sessions included domestic violence, shifting spousal relationships, and the developmental and emotional needs of children in new cultural environments.

These forums provided space for parents to speak freely about their views and experiences. For example, equalitarian relationships characteristic of American families produced tensions in spousal and parent/child interpersonal relations for immigrant families from cultures based in traditional gender role expectations. The American "progressive" approach to education was not favored by most parents who were more comfortable with formal models of structured classrooms with teachers in authoritative roles.

Some parents were concerned with supporting children's acculturation while helping them maintain suitable personal and group identification with the norms and traditions of their native cultures. Nearly all parents worried about children becoming "Americanized" and socialized into a youth culture that encourages behaviors that are unacceptable in their native cultures.

Client engagement was influenced by the perception on the part of some families that contacts with service providers would be problem-focused or biased against them because of their immigrant status. Parents failed to keep school appointments not because of a lack of interest in the progress of children, but because they felt school officials did not always forthrightly deal with concerns about their children being "picked on" by peers, or being treated differently by some teachers. While some parents persisted in the face of perceived unfair treatment and discrimination, others were resentful and were discouraged from seeking assistance from provider agencies. Some expressed concerns about "No Child Left Behind" policies requiring children for whom English was not their primary language, to take standardized tests in English within a specified timeframe of arriving in the country. Few, if any, had favorable thoughts about Children's Services, with most feeling that involvement with the agency would result in the removal of their children.

Student-Learning Contracts and Portfolios

Student-learning contracts and portfolios were used to strengthen the integration of learning in class and field, and supplement process recordings as the traditional field education-teaching tool. These instruments focused on knowledge, values, and skills required for development of advanced concentration field practica competencies, and the educational objectives of ICWFP. This formal documentation made it possible for students to retrospectively review the evolution of their professional thinking and how they were growing in practice competencies and personal development.

Learning contracts were prepared by students with input from field instructors and faculty advisors. They were reviewed to identify assets and learning needs and modified to shape assignments as needed. Students were given more discretion in preparing portfolios, making entries as frequently as they chose with a minimum requirement of once each week. The portfolios encouraged a focus on macro level issues that had implications for direct practice and service outcomes. This individualized approach was intended to support critical thinking, problem solving, and "thinking outside of the box." Reflective thinking and focus on macro level systems proved especially useful for surfacing ethical dilemmas emerging in case practice and for examining applicability of intervention models and practice theories anchored in Western conceptualizations of health and wellness. The portfolios effectively linked "case to cause" and were useful for developing monthly clinical consultation agendas.

The qualitative analysis of student portfolios and learning contracts is organized under several themes. These themes include: integration of knowledge, values and skills in practice; development of professional identity and differential practice approaches; skill development for best clinical practices with immigrant families; and integration of ICWFP guiding principles in practice.

The structure of neighborhood-based field education units proved to be an essential ingredient for achieving the integration of knowledge, values, and skills essential for providing culturally competent services to immigrant families in practice. This structure contributed to an *esprit de corps* among students that supported a strong professional perspective and identification with the professional role. This structure provided peer support and group sharing that assisted students coping with the frustrations of new program start-up, difficulties in engaging the target immigrant families, and new insights into the challenges of implementing new programs across complex bureaucratic systems.

> At this point, everyone was frustrated about why finding cases became difficult … I understood why it was a hardship. It was frustrating to see how things were playing out but it was expected. Mid-terms were coming up … so it was a time when my stress level was high. I really felt bad for [those without adequate cases] and thought more about the program in depth. I started thinking about the program and how it could be improved.… There was definitely a lot I learned in reference to program development.

By mid-semester, student reflections indicated new understandings of the policy and organizational context for direct practice; they developed insights into barriers to engagement that resulted from both organizational arrangements of the host agency and client "resistances."

> During the later part of December through January I have learned that I need to be patient when it comes to working in organizations where policies and red tape can dominate and hinder progress. I am learning to accept things I cannot change … I am discovering the difficulty that teachers can have controlling the classroom. I am also learning that when I meet with African families to discuss the conduct of their children they point to the teacher and the school as the source of the problem. I am attempting to work with families at identifying how together we can work on their children's conduct and academics. However, there appears to be a certain level of non-receptivity on the part of families.

DEVELOPMENT OF PROFESSIONAL IDENTITY AND DIFFERENTIAL
PRACTICE APPROACHES

Students in the advanced concentrations typically begin to articulate a greater degree of comfort in their professional role, a growing sense of self-efficacy, and an increasing range of professional competencies. These were difficult tasks for students to achieve within the context of a developing project. Students assigned to the Children's Services agency-based unit faced the added challenge of accomplishing these learning tasks while confronting dilemmas inherent to professional practice in bureaucratic settings, and balancing the sometimes competing value orientations of the profession and the protective/investigatory function of the agency. The unfolding of this process is illuminated in portfolio entries where power imbalances inherent to the worker–client relationship and meaning of the client's rights for self-determination are discussed.

> This new role as a social work intern/fellow made me somewhat uncomfortable in my interaction with my client ... I had to tune into my feelings with Ms. X throughout our session, while in my child protective role I was not predominately focused on feelings. I also had to be cognizant of my professional use of self and stay where Ms. X was ... Nonetheless I learnt how to share the power ... and I am beginning to interact with her from a social work—as opposed to an investigatory—standpoint.

> I had to learn not to see the case as an investigation ... get into my own feelings and stay on the right path. There were some non-verbal cues used by the client that I realized and I asked about them. In the past, I would have said "she has an attitude, and I am not going to deal with that." Now I ... work to explore non-verbal (communication) more.

SKILL DEVELOPMENT FOR BEST CLINICAL PRACTICES WITH
IMMIGRANT FAMILIES

The need for a mix of concrete and mental health services was evident in the presenting problems of families. For example, clients experienced a range of problems including the loss of family members, domestic violence, homelessness, loss of status and income, poverty, discrimination, and marginalization. Many of the families emigrated from countries where extreme poverty and political unrest were not uncommon. For some, as reported in parent seminars, their children's adjustment experiences surfaced unresolved feelings as they recalled their own experiences of loneliness, social isolation, alienation, and peer rejection upon initial arrival in the United States.

The following narratives highlight opportunities for teaching practice competencies for conducting culturally competent assessments that address psychosocial needs. They provide a glimpse into the student's awareness of the immigration experience and call for supervisory time to address the import of their impact on work with immigrant families.

> I accompanied my family's caretaker to the Children's Services housing subsidy unit ... The paperwork was picked up and an appointment was done for that same Thursday. On our way back she told me about the horrors about coming to the U.S. We arrived to her home where we filled out the paper work and left everything ready for the following appointment.

> A majority of the new immigrants feel that resettlement means starting a new life—a career, a family and becoming part of a new community ... some still try to cope with memories of violence and pain of losing friends and family members.

Expectations of field-education curriculum in the direct service concentration are for students to conduct clinically focused assessments from which appropriate therapeutic interventions are formulated; and to recognize and explore taboo and emotionally charged material. A paradoxical finding revealed that, despite evidence of client need and student interests, most case activities involved information, referral, and helping clients obtain concrete services—despite clear emotional components also needing attention.

> I visited another family in Chinatown; the father of the family appeared depressed, angry, and helpless. He stated he was not familiar with the family court system about his rights and tried to seek help for his girlfriend to parental counseling. In addition, he is having problems seeking legal assistance due to financial issues.

In attempting to understand the skewing of case activities towards the provision of concrete and information and referral services, the researchers hypothesized that the highly politicized context of immigration policy may have inhibited dialogue or contributed to student reluctance to bring up emotionally charged issues for fear of being misunderstood or being "politically incorrect." This speculation is supported by the following entry expressing concern about perceived parental overuse of physical discipline with children:

> It's difficult to bring it up with them, and I feel uncomfortable broaching the concept of reinforcement—hitting someone as punishment for fighting—this is not good role modeling.

Some students found it especially challenging to demonstrate nonjudgmental attitudes around more emotionally laden customs and practices. In addition to being difficult areas for the student to explore, families themselves may have been reluctant to disclose information around certain practices that are significantly different from American norms and customs. While these observations are speculative, findings suggest that students are in need of additional educational supports to meet learning requirements of advanced concentration field education and to develop skills for the exploration of emotionally laden content with immigrant families from non-Western countries whose customs and beliefs are significantly different from their own.

INTEGRATING ICWFP GUIDING PRINCIPLES INTO PRACTICE

Ecological Perspective

Portfolio entries illustrate student integration and application of the ecological perspective. This perspective is observed through their assessment of multiple systems affecting family stability; their consideration of the implications of culture in understanding client presenting problems and in planning interventions; and their increasing understanding of organizational contexts and the implications of culturally inadequate policies common to systems that have yet to accommodate to the needs of immigrant families.

> As a child protective worker … of seven years, I worked with children and families, but the focus was on the children. The families … were not limited to immigrant families. The difference with this program is that my caseload is going to be immigrant families from around the world. I will be assessing the organizational, political and cultural environments.

> We spoke some about the Board of Education and the inane protocols in the 'No Child Left Behind' bill. Every immigrant student is required to take the same [standardized] test as native English speakers after they have been in this country 10 months. Many immigrant parents do not understand this and thus are unprepared. So one of the services we could offer could be a group for parents helping them to understand the educational system.

Strengths-Based Perspective and Family-Centered Practice

Strengths-based perspectives and family-centered practice are reflected in the following narrative where the student contemplates a change in previously held notions about best practices with immigrant families. The narrative gives some indication of critical thinking related to the development of an individualized approach to practice that is child-centered while considering the family's total needs.

> As a caseworker, for Children's Services for more than six years, my primary concern is with children and their well-being. Consequently regardless of the circumstances surrounding immigrant families, I tend to focus on what is best for the children. This has often forced me to overlook my personal feelings about the adults or their plight, whatever that might be. However, I am not sure that I am completely objective in my assessment of any given situation and, consequently, I am not sure whether I consistently offer the best solution. A learning need is to learn to objectively assess immigrant families so I can provide assistance that is best suited for the family.

Culturally Competent Practice

Portfolios were especially helpful in strengthening teaching opportunities for culturally competent practice with new immigrants. They revealed challenging experiences that exacerbated feelings of difference, and for some promoted feelings of cultural shock.

> ... is very different from any school I ever went to—or set foot in, for that matter. It's louder, more out of control and uglier. The building is pretty grim and unpleasant. Some of the kids are large for their grade—I wonder if they stayed back multiple times? Or perhaps they are just big ... the buildings are ugly, especially the large public housing projects. The neighborhood feels isolated, an island at the end of the line ... I initially thought X [another community school] was pretty awful, but now it looks like a country club to me!

On the other hand, the existent world views of some students enabled them to comfortably incorporate content from the enhanced educational programs as they prepared for encounters with culturally different families.

> Attending the orientation and reading the articles distributed, I realized that interventions tested on one group may not fit the cultural framework of others ... One of my assets I can bring to this project is sharing my understanding of cultural difference between the U.S. (Western Perspective) culture and my culture ...

The following narratives illustrate developing culturally competent practice skills and reflections on factors influencing engagement and the quality of the worker–client relationship. They also illustrate movement from a "one-size-fits-all" approach to an appreciation for diversity and the implications of these differences for individualized assessments and the differential use-of-self.

> I will respect the immigrant's culture and community. Hence, this will help me to learn more about their strengths and resources and understand the context of the families' needs so that I can develop service plans that preserve the families. As a bi-lingual intern, I can help immigrant families understand the developmental needs of their children and (appropriate) disciplinary approaches.

> I am also learning that there appears to be a distinct difference in the way Hispanic families respond to me vs. African families. I am finding it more difficult to engage African families.... I am attempting to work with the families at identifying how together we can work on their children's conduct and academics. However, there appears to be a certain level of non-receptivity on the part of families.

The following student illustrates ongoing development of insights about informal patterns of service utilization and help-seeking behaviors of different immigrant groups useful for teaching concepts around social capital development in immigrant communities.

> I am discovering that African families in East Harlem all know each other. They seem to be a part of a little village. However, it is not clear to me yet how they help each other. For example, when completing a Section 8 application for one of my families, I asked the mother to provide the name of a person who could be listed as an emergency contact—a friend or neighbor. The mother was not able to name anyone. Yet, when I named various families ... the mother knew them all.

The following narrative highlights challenges faced in teaching cultural competent practice when belief systems support behaviors that are significantly different from those supported by the socialization experiences of the novice student.

> I met with the family of a newly referred child—the wife and son have only been here a few months—if we hadn't done all this work on cultural difference I might have thought there was something wrong in the marital relationship—the wife was completely silent, kept her eyes on the ground, and walked about seven feet behind her husband ... It may be cultural difference, but I still don't like it!

These narratives underscore the importance of creating safe learning environments to non-defensively examine existent world views and personal biases. Anchoring diversity dialogues with students in the ethical guidelines of the profession versus personal value preferences and beliefs was essential for a productive non-defensive examination of the profession's historic commitment to diversity and social justice. Discussions of this nature are likely to become commonplace in class and field in light of the increasing global context of practice.

IMPLICATIONS FOR MODEL BUILDING

Criteria for Student Selection

Attributes found to facilitate a "good fit" for integrating learning goals of the educational model included an ability to draw upon a broad repertoire of theoretical frameworks for assessing client needs, and developing practice interventions and a strong sense of social justice. Other strengths and skill sets supporting the integration of leaning goals were a willingness to examine pre-existing ethnocentric world views and an appreciation for the constraints of professional practice in bureaucratic settings. Critical thinking was essential in examining universal applicability of theories based in a Western conceptualization of health and wellness.

These observations are similar to literature findings relative to teaching skills for culturally competent social work practice cited earlier (Devore & Schlesinger 1996), and those suggesting that many students are not aware of their personal biases or how these influence their perceptions and attitudes in practice (Colvin-Burque, Zugazaga, & Davis-Maye, 2007; Hepworth, Rooney, & Larsen, 2002). This underscores ICWFP findings that a pre-requisite for practice with immigrant families is a willingness to examine ethnocentric worldviews. This finding has implications for social work education and faculty supports provided to students, and point to essential foci for first year content and experiences.

The analysis of the pre–post-test scores and portfolio entries revealed that as the academic year progressed, students moved toward a more re-alistic assessment of their level of cultural competence. Further, enhanced by interactions with a diverse peer group—including ethnicity, race, lan-guage, and national origin—there was a greater willingness to give up well-intentioned notions of a color-blind society. Non-threatening interactions with a supportive peer group undoubtedly played a role in an increased readiness for adoption of social work's multicultural perspective affirming the value of diverse populations. The ability of students to demonstrate this kind of transition in their thinking was supported by their ability to draw on personal family histories of immigration and cultural roots. Students who were first or second generation immigrants themselves were especially sensitive to Eurocentric world views that can potentially constrain effective practice with immigrant populations, which is illustrated in the following student narrative.

> The fellows might take a certain view as a universal perspective, which is actually an internalized Western perspective. Sharing my cultural perspec-tive ... may change their assuming as universal, the Western perspective.

Structuring Field Education Experiences

Reisch and Jarman-Rohde (2000) in a discussion of contemporary societal trends that are changing the character of American society, encourage social work educators to bring the classroom to the community. Focusing on the implications of these changes for field education curriculum, these authors argue that school–agency partnerships offer benefits of involving students and constituents in defining community needs and evaluating the effective-ness of agency programs for the context of today's practice environment.

As illustrated in student narratives, community-based field education units provide a wealth of opportunities for developing cross-curriculum assignments. For example, community-mapping assignments assisted students' identification of formal and informal helping systems in catchment neighborhoods, which supported learning objectives of the practice and research curriculum. Students were also better able to integrate policy content as parents reported similar experiences about the impact of policies of the host agencies on their aspirations for the "American Dream," or for diminishing or increasing access to essential family support services. The integration of content from human behavior was strengthened by the immersion in the community since students were better able to make the link between community conditions and client outcomes, and the interrelatedness of "personal troubles and public issues." Importantly, the community-based structure encouraged a more balanced view for understanding individual and societal responsibility in causal attributions. For immigrant populations there has been a tendency to attribute causation of child maltreatment to the lack of acculturation or cultural norms and practices that contribute to aberrant parental behaviors that place children at risk. Being both *in* the community and *of* the community, promoted a balanced view about the role of personal and institutional responsibility for understanding causal linkages of child abuse and neglect, thus contributing to an appreciation for social work's role of advocacy in child welfare.

The Added Value of Learning Portfolios as a Teaching Tool

Portfolios are an effective tool for teaching knowledge, values and skills integral to the field education curricula (Cournoyer & Stanley, 2002), and for promoting diversity-learning goals integral to the project. When used in conjunction with process recordings, an added value of portfolios is that attention is drawn away from the exclusive focus on the interaction with individual clients, thus making it possible for a closer examination of the larger context of practice influencing both student learning and client outcomes. Further, student reflective thinking in portfolio narratives identified rich teaching opportunities for integrating core content across curriculum areas, supporting critical thinking and analytical skills essential for understanding the impact of institutional structures on the creation of social problems endemic to certain populations and implications for direct practice (Schatz, 2004). These observations are similar to study findings on the effectiveness of learning portfolios for achieving goals of social work education. Portfolios were found to have added advantages of enabling an objective review of student achievement of learning objectives, practice competencies, and examination of achieving the integration of theory and practice. Additional implications exist for training field instructors and the need to increase their ability to incorporate broader social justice perspectives into their teaching responsibilities.

Strengthening Multicultural Content

There is continued discourse among social work educators as to whether multicultural content is best taught as specialized course offerings or infused throughout the curriculum (Atherton, & Bolland, 1997; Chestang, 1988). The project experience indicates that whichever approach is taken, traditional approaches must be complimented by new strategies essential for expanding the knowledge base and increasing awareness to prepare graduates for the demands of practice in a global environment that raise difficult issues of practice and professional ethics.

ICWFP first year findings underscore the need for strengthening diversity content in consideration of the increasing global context within which social work graduates will practice. An assumption of the ICWFP was that students selected for the project had successfully mastered the content of the professional foundation. However, a consistent appraisal of students was that their exposure to diversity content in the professional foundation year in class or field was insufficient to support a knowledge base for understanding the problems and needs of new immigrants.

CONCLUSIONS

Year one of the ICWFP experience illustrates many benefits of university– public child welfare agency partnerships for the planning and design of educational and program innovations that keep pace with the changing demands of the child welfare practice context and emerging new needs of children and families. The ICWFP enjoyed the benefits that come with expanding this traditional partnership to include community-based agencies committed to adapting existing programs to meet the needs of new immigrants.

The findings reported underscore the many educational benefits accrued from the structure of community-based field education units, the center-piece of the educational model, that bring students in closer interaction with immigrant communities and provider agencies. The community-based model provided rich opportunities for teaching and learning of multicultural content. Joining students placed within the public child welfare agency unit with students placed within the neighborhood school and community hospital in seminars, learning activities, and discussions of program planning enhanced their appreciation of the commonalities of public and private sector child welfare community practice.

In addition, the community-based model allowed for the incorporation of concepts from service learning, a pedagogical approach that integrates community service with academic study as a means for encouraging critical thinking, reflection, and creative problem solving (Lemieux & Allen, 2007). The ICWFP expanded the traditional field education model that develops student assignments around the needs of the placement agencies and academic requirements of the school, to formulate assignments around the needs of target immigrant communities as they evolved from interactions with provider agencies and families. As illustrated in the discussion of qualitative findings from portfolios and learning contracts, these tools were highly successful in encouraging student critical thinking and self-reflection that enhanced the achievement of educational goals.

Although the benefits are substantial, challenges of these organizational alliances are those related to consensus building activities required to codify the interests of the participating organizations into a cohesive strategy for achieving common goals while advancing their individual missions. Further, the ICWFP experience indicated that time constraints of the academic calendar imposed a structure onto these dialogues which sometimes appeared insensitive to the time normally required for such complex organizational negotiations to evolve.

As the ICWFP moves towards institutional status, the project will be housed at the New York University School of Social Work, McSilver Institute for Poverty Policy Research. This placement will allow for sustaining and expanding ICWFP core objectives through the integration with current institute research projects examining the multiple dimensions of poverty and its impact on many client populations. This integration will strengthen the research capability of the ICWFP and open new opportunities for longitudinal and evaluation studies that contribute to empirically-based knowledge for identifying promising best practices and competencies needed for effective interventions with immigrant children and their families in child welfare and related fields of practice.

REFERENCES

Administration for Children's Services (ACS). (2007). *Improved outcomes for children: The second phase of ACS' action plan for child safety.* New York, NY: Author.

Atherton, C. R., & Bolland, K. A. (1997). The multiculturalism debate and social work education: A response to Van Soest. *Journal of Social Work Education, 33,* 123–150.

Balgopal, P. R. (2000). *Social work practice with immigrant and refugees.* New York, NY: Colombia University Press.

Belanger, K., Bullard, L. B., & Green, D. K. (Eds.) (2008). Special issue: Racial disproportionality in child welfare. *Child Welfare, 87*(2).

Browne, C., & Mills, C. (2001). Theoretical frameworks: Ecological model strengths perspective, and empowerment theory. In R. Fong & S. Furuto (Eds.), *Culturally competent practice: Skills, intervention, and evaluations*, (pp. 10–32). Needham Heights, MA: Allyn and Bacon.

Capps, R. (1999). *Hardships among children of immigrants. Findings from the 1999 National Survey of American Families*. Retrieved from http://www.urban.org/publications/310096.html

Carten, A. J., & Dumpson, J. R. (2004). Family preservation and neighborhood–based services: An Africentric perspective. In Everett, J., Chipungu. S. P. & Leashore, B. R. (Eds.), *Child welfare revisited* (pp. 225–241). New Brunswick, New Jersey: Rutgers University Press.

Carten, A. J., & Finch, J. B. (1998). *Evaluation and enhancement of child welfare field placement* [unpublished report]. New York, NY: Social Work Education Consortium.

Carten, A, J., & Goodman, H. (2005). An educational model for child welfare practice with Anglophone Caribbean families. *Child Welfare, 84,* 771–790.

Chahine, Z., & van Straaten, J. (2005). Serving immigrant families and children in New York City's child welfare system. *Child Welfare, 84,* 713–723.

Chestang, L. W. (1988). Infusion of minority content in the curriculum. In D. Jacobs & D. D. Bowles (Eds.), *Ethnicity and race* (pp. 230–240). Silver Spring, MD: NASW Press.

Council on Social Work Education (CSWE). (2003). *Handbook of Accreditation Standards and Procedures* (5th ed.) Alexandra, VA: Author.

Colvin–Burque, A., Zugazaga, C. B., & Davis–Maye, D. (2007). Can cultural competency be taught? Evaluating the impact of the SOAP model. *Journal of Social Work Education, 43,* 223–241.

Cournoyer, B., & Stanley, M. (2002). *The social work portfolio: Planning, assessing and documenting lifelong learning in a dynamic profession*. Pacific Grove, CA: Brooks/Cole Thompson Learning.

Devore, W., & Schlesinger, E. G. (1996). *Ethnic-sensitive social work practice* (4th edition). St. Louis, MO: Mosby.

Drachman, D. (1992). A stage-of-migration framework for services to immigrant populations. *Social Work, 37,* 68–72.

Everette, J., Chipungu, S., & Leashore, B. (Eds.) (2004). *Child welfare revisited: An Afrocentric perspective*. New Brunswick, NJ: Rutgers University Press.

Earner, I., & Rivera, H. (Eds.) (2005). Special issue: Immigrants and refugees in child welfare. *Child Welfare, 84*(5).

Fellin, P. (2000). Revisiting multiculturalism in social work. *Journal of Social Work Education, 36,* 261–278.

Francs, A. E. (2000). Social work practice with African–descent immigrants. In P. R. Balgopal (Ed.), *Social work practice with immigrant and refugees* (pp. 127–166). New York, NY: Colombia University Press.

Franzosi, R. (2008). *Content analysis. Volume I.* Thousand Oaks, CA: Sage Benchmarks in Social Research Methods Series.

Furuto, S. B. C. L. (2004). Theoretical perspectives for culturally competent with immigrant children and families. In R. Fong (Ed.), *Culturally competent practice with immigrant and refugee children and families* (pp. 19–38). New York, NY: Guildford Press.

Hepworth, D. H., Rooney, R. H., & Larson, J. (2002). *Direct social work practice: Theory and skills* (6th ed.). Pacific Grove, CA: Brooks/Cole.

Hill, R. B. (2006). *Synthesis of research on disproportionality in child welfare. An update.* Washington, DC: Center for the Study of Social Policy.

Holden, G., Meenaghan, T., Anastas, J. & Metrey, G. (2002). Outcomes of social work education: The case for social work self–efficacy. *Journal of Social Work Education, 38,* 115–133.

Immigrant Child Welfare Fellowship Project. (2008). *Children of the world community program: Implementation report. 2006–2007.* New York, NY: New York City Social Work Education Consortium.

Lemieux, C. M., & Allen, P. V. (2007). Service learning in social work education: The state of knowledge, pedagogical practicalities and practice conundrums. *Journal of Social Work Education, 43,* 309–325.

Lincroft, Y., Resner, J., Leung, & Bussiere, A. (2006). *Undercounted. Underserved: Immigrant and refugee families in the child welfare system.* Baltimore, MD: Annie Casey Foundation.

Lum, D., & Lu, Y. E. (2007). Skill development. In D. Lum (Ed.), *Culturally competent practice: A framework for understanding diverse groups and justice issues* (3rd ed.) (pp. 185–225). Belmont, CA: Thomson Brooks Cole.

Mattingly, J. (2005). *Enormous strides for NYC children and families.* New York, NY: National Association of Social Workers.

McRoy, R. (2002, April). Over–representation of children of color in the child welfare system. Paper presented at the Child Welfare Lecture Series, Hunter College School of Social Work, National Resource Center for Foster Care and Permanency Planning.

Nash, K. A., & Velazquez, J. (2003). *Cultural competence: A guide for human service agencies.* Washington, DC: Child Welfare League of America Press.

National Association of Social Workers (NASW). (2001). *NASW standards for cultural competency in social work practice.* Washington, DC: Author.

Passel, J. S., & Suro, R. (2005). *Rise, peak and decline: Trends in U.S. immigration 1992–2004.* Washington, DC: Pew Hispanic Center.

Pine, B. A., & Drachman, D. (2005). Effective child welfare practice with immigrant and refugee children and their families. *Child Welfare, 84,* 537–562.

Ponterroto, J. G., Gretchen, D., Utsey, S. O., Riger, B. P., & Austin, R. (2002). A revision of the multicultural counseling awareness scale. *Journal of Multicultural Counseling and Development, 30,* 153–181.

Potocky-Tripodi, M. (2002). *Best practices for social work practice with refugees and immigrants.* New York, NY: Columbia University Press.

Reisch, M., & Jarman-Rohde, L (2000). The future of social work in the United States. Implications for field education. *Journal of Social Work Education, 36,* 201–214.

Roberts, D. (2002). *Shattered Bonds: The color of child welfare.* New York, NY: Basic Books.

Salvo, J. (2005). *Immigrant New York in the millennium.* New York, NY: Mayor's Office of City Planning, Population Division.

Samantrai, K. (2004). *Culturally competent public child welfare practice.* Pacific Grove, CA: Thomson, Brooks/Cole.

Schatz, M. (2004). Using portfolios: Integrating learning and promoting reflections through portfolios for social work students. *Advances in Social Work, 5*(1), 105–123.

Urban Institute (2002). *Immigrant Well-Being in New York and Los Angeles.* Retrieved from http://www.urban.org/UploadedPDF/310566_ImmigrantWell Being.pdf

Index

Page numbers in *Italics* represent tables.
Page numbers in **Bold** represent figures.